Outwitting Back Pain

Outwitting Back Pain

Why Your Lower Back Hurts and How to Make It Stop

Ellis F. Friedman, M.D.

with Abbi Perets

Series Concept Created by Bill Adler Jr.

THE LYONS PRESS
Guilford, Connecticut

An imprint of The Globe Pequot Press

The Lyons Press is an imprint of The Globe Pequot Press.

10 9 8 7 6 5 4 3 2 1

Printed in the United States of America

Book design by Stephanie Doyle

ISBN 1-59228-432-9

Library of Congress Cataloging-in-Publication Data is available on file.

Contents

List of Illustrations

Preface

I lived in Berks County, Pennsylvania, from the day I was born until I retired after twenty-eight years of working as an orthopaedic surgeon. Berks County is in southeastern Pennsylvania, smack dab in the heart of the Pennsylvania Dutch country, where people say things like, "Throw the cow over the fence some hay," and, "Outen the lights."

In 1967, I was a brand-new first-year resident in orthopaedic surgery at The Reading Hospital. My patient, a delightful farm woman, had an abnormality of one of the bones in her lower spine. Now, on any side-view x-ray of this bone, some parts look like a Scottie dog with its ear, eye, nose, foreleg, and body. If the "Scottie dog" has a "broken neck," then the patient has a condition that needs surgery.

I began to take the patient's history, asking her, "What brings you here to the hospital?"

She innocently replied, "Why, my doctor told me I have doggy trouble . . . but we don't have any doggies at home, just cows and pigs!"

Apparently, animals figure prominently in discussing back injuries in the Pennsylvania Dutch country. When I lectured on back problems to the student nurses at The Reading Hospital and Medical Center, my presentation was titled "The Birdies of Berks County."

I told the student nurses that the birds of Berks County were capable of causing terrible back problems. These birds, in fact, were undoubtedly as vicious as those in the classic Alfred Hitchcock film *The Birds*. I knew this, I explained, because I'd seen many Pennsylvania Dutch patients over the years, who always came in with the same complaint,

"I was bending over, and all of a sudden it flew in my back, and it flew down my leg!"

That's actually a succinct and accurate description of how some back problems begin: a sudden, sharp pain in the low back that then radiates down the leg. The cause? Well, that's not necessarily so simple. Some kinds of back pain can be outwitted with a quick and easy fix. Other times, the same kind of pain in the same general area can be caused by much more complex problems—requiring special diagnostic tests and, possibly, surgery. Outwitting such pain takes more knowledge and skill, but it can often be done.

In this book, I'm going to help you to learn about the back: what it is, how it works, why good backs go bad, how we figure that out, and what we can do about it. I promise that if I have to use a fancy medical term, I'll immediately define it in lay language. Each chapter will build on what you've learned in the preceding one.

One feature of this book needs to be explained here. I refer to doctors using the masculine *he*. I have been happily married for thirty years to a wonderful woman who, even before we were wed, raised my consciousness about gender neutrality. I seriously considered always saying *he or she* in this book, but even my wife felt that it was unnecessary in this case and said she would not be offended. Believe me, some of the best doctors I know are women!

There are a number of people whom I must thank for their invaluable help. Each of them kindly took time out of a busy schedule to provide me with important materials. Dr. Irving Ehrlich, chief of radiology at St. Joseph's Hospital, Reading, Pennsylvania, sent me MRI scans and CAT scans. Dr. Randall Winn, chief of the Section of Nuclear Medicine at The Reading Hospital and Medical Center in Reading, Pennsylvania, provided the bone scans. Dr. Mihra Taljanovic, assistant professor of clinical radiology, University of Arizona Health Sciences Center, provided myelograms and other films. Dr. Jeffrey Lisse, professor of medicine and director of the Arizona Arthritis Center Osteoporosis Program at the University of Arizona—and my neighbor—provided technical expertise. Dr. John Bower, who delivered our kids and is a life-long friend, and his wife, Jill, a certified nurse practitioner in ob-gyn, read chapter 8 and made excellent suggestions.

Bill Adler, of Adler & Robin Books, originated the "Outwitting . . ." series, and I'm grateful to him for encouraging me and for being my agent. Lilly Golden, my editor at Lyons Press, was a delight to work with and made the publishing process a lot of fun.

My son, Lex, the esoteric grammar maven, and my daughter, Marnie, the careful reader, both made excellent suggestions for improving readability. My wife, Irene, gave me enormous encouragement; in addition, she's the world's best proofreader. She, too, offered many ideas for clarifying concepts, and I can't thank her enough for all her love and support.

Finally, I thank my daughter, Abbi, who's responsible for urging me to write about how back pain is treated, and who got me into this in the first place. She meticulously reviewed every chapter and "Abbified" it, making changes that transformed the layout and made the book so good. And she did it with such ease!

I hope that you find this book to be helpful and that you enjoy reading it as much as I've enjoyed writing it.

Introduction

If you've ever suffered from back pain, you know just how much you want to outwit it. And if misery really does love company, you've got plenty. Back pain is a huge cause of temporary impairment in the United States.

✦ Each year, about 10 percent of the population of the United States suffers at least one episode of lower back pain.

✦ Eighty percent of adults will experience lower back pain at some point during their lifetimes.

✦ Up to 20 percent of working people experience back pain each year.

✦ Spinal diseases are *the most common cause of disability for adults under age forty-five.*

✦ At any given time, about 1 percent of the U.S. population is temporarily disabled because of back pain.

✦ Lower back pain is the second leading cause of absenteeism at work in the United States and *results in more lost productivity than any other medical problem.*

✦ Low back problems are the most frequent reason for referral to orthopaedic surgeons, neurosurgeons, and physicians specializing in occupational medicine.

✦ Two and a half million patients see doctors each year because of low back complaints.

✦ Lower back pain is the leading workers' compensation problem.

✦ Each year, low back complaints result in *$15 billion in lost wages.*

✦ Seventeen million people are on either permanent or temporary disability because of low back problems.

✦ Ten million workers have functional limitations as a result of lower back pain.

Outwitting Back Pain will teach you why you have developed lower back pain and how you can try to get better. This book won't belittle you by suggesting that your pain is caused by tension or that it can be cured by following one specific set of exercises. Instead, *Outwitting Back Pain* will offer you a chance to understand the structure and function of the back; knowing that, you'll learn how the back can be injured. Then you'll find out how problems can be diagnosed; after that, you'll learn the methods of treatment.

This book will give you practical information that you can begin to use immediately, as well as the knowledge and confidence you need to speak effectively with doctors and other caregivers in the long term. Doctors love to use big words, and you're about to see that the vocabulary of orthopaedics is filled with them. All the important terms here are in **boldface** so you can pinpoint them easily. I've tried to demystify them by defining them in lay language, so now you'll know some of medicine's secrets. For a quick reference, these terms are listed again in the glossary at the end. I give the lay synonym each time I use a medical term, so you won't have to hunt through previous chapters to find its meaning.

I've used many photographs of x-rays in this book because one picture really is worth a thousand words. Most of these x-rays came from my own personal collection. These x-ray films illustrate the various conditions I'll be describing, so to make them worthwhile, I've tried to make you radiologists-for-a-day in one easy lesson by doing two things:

1. Accompanying each x-ray is a labeled outline drawing of that x-ray. This should make it much easier to understand exactly what the x-ray shows.

2. Below every x-ray is a box labeled X-ray Vision. You don't need to read it in order to understand what the x-ray is showing. It contains more detailed information about the various things that can be seen on the x-ray, and it is for readers who enjoy a detailed, technical explanation.

Back pain, as you're about to see, isn't just due to one condition. It occurs because of some kind of problem involving bones, joints, muscles, ligaments, discs, or nerves—or some combination of them. It's time now to start learning about back pain, because the sooner you do, the sooner you can get better.

Chapter One

THE BACK
WHAT IT IS AND HOW IT WORKS

In order to understand how the back can be injured and how those injuries can be diagnosed and treated, first you need to learn about the spine itself. Once you know what makes up the spine and how its parts function, then it will be easy to see what happens when things go wrong. You'll also be able to use your knowledge of the structure and function of the spine to recognize why and how various treatments may help correct back and neck problems.

There's a lot to learn in this chapter, and the material isn't easy. But if you've been suffering back pain for any amount of time, it's worth reading carefully. I won't test you, and I can't tell if your eyes are glazing over the way my children's do when I "talk doctor" to them. But trust me: If you tough it out through this chapter, the rest will be much easier—and will help you treat your back pain more effectively.

The Spinal Column

The spine, or, more simply, "the back," consists of thirty-three bones, twenty-eight of which are separate and five of which are solidly joined together. (**Fig. 1–1**)

Figure 1 - 1

The Spinal Column

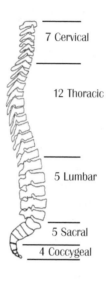

7 Cervical

12 Thoracic

5 Lumbar

5 Sacral

4 Coccygeal

Latin Lesson

In medicine, we always try to be fancy, and we frequently say things in a fancy way because it makes us look very learned to our patients. So we don't call them "back bones"; instead, each bone of the spine is called a **vertebra. (Fig. 1– 2A, B)** Vertebra is a nice, fancy Latin word; it's a feminine Latin noun, so the plural is vertebrae.

Figure 1-2

A Lumbar Vertebra

S = Spinous process
T = Transverse process
L = Lamina
P = Pedicle
F = Facet
B = Body

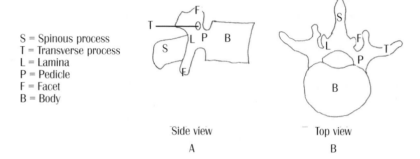

Side view · · · · · · · · · · · · · · · Top view
A · B

Your neck has seven bones—**cervical vertebrae**. Beneath them, your ribs attach to twelve upper-mid back bones called **thoracic vertebrae**. Under these are the five lower back bones called **lumbar vertebrae**, as well as a group of five bones at the base of the spine that are fused together into one big, solid, bony anchor called the **sacrum**. Actually, four tailbones called the **coccyx** sit below the sacrum, but they are left over from evolution eons ago and have no function. (Just because the coccyx has no real purpose doesn't mean it can't cause lots of pain, though. It can—and I'll talk about why later on.) If you look at a normal spine from the front or from behind, it is perfectly straight from the neck to the tailbone. (**Fig. 1–3A**)

If you look at the spine from behind and you see a C-shaped (**Fig. 1–3B**) or S-shaped curve, (**Fig. 1–3C**) that's abnormal and is called **scoliosis**, or curvature of the spine.

Figure 1-3

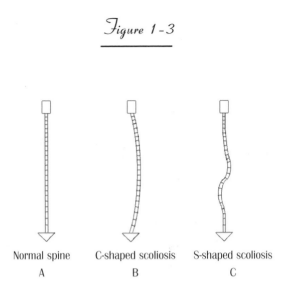

Normal spine	C-shaped scoliosis	S-shaped scoliosis
A	B	C

When you look at the spine from the side, you see a series of gentle curves. In the neck, or cervical, spine, there is a C-shaped curve (called **lordosis**) in which the midpart of the C faces toward the front. In the upper-mid back, or thoracic, spine is another C-shaped curve, but the midpart of this curve faces toward the rear and is called **kyphosis**. In the lower back, or lumbar spine, is yet another C-shaped curve facing toward the front; again, this is called **lordosis**. Of course, we can be fancy and refer to a lordotic curve or a kyphotic curve. (**Fig. 1–4**)

An excessive amount of kyphosis in the midback region—especially in the upper part of that area—causes what's commonly referred to as a hunchback. An excessive lordotic curve in the low back is often called a swayback. And if the low back has lost its lordotic curve, people call that a poker spine.

Figure 1-4

Lordosis and Kyphosis

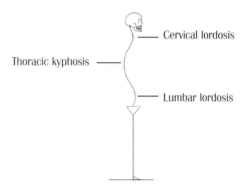

Cervical lordosis

Thoracic kyphosis

Lumbar lordosis

The Parts of a Vertebra

It might help to imagine the spine—or the spinal column, or the twenty-four vertebrae of the neck, midback, and lumbar spine—as a series of row houses. A row house usually contains a basement, walls, a roof, eaves and gutters, and a chimney. Each row house is connected to the next, and each row house provides a nice, comfortable home for the people who live inside. (**Fig. 1–5**)

The vertebrae also provide a nice, comfortable home for the structures that "live" inside them: the spinal cord and the spinal nerve roots. A vertebra has several parts. You've already seen fancy drawings of how a vertebra actually looks from the side and top. From now on, the drawings here will be less fancy for two reasons:

1. You don't really need to know every specialized bony projection or surface.

2. It's much easier to learn from drawings similar to those on a blue-print, with front, side, and top views. (**Fig. 1–6 A, B, C**)

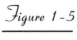

Figure 1 - 5

A Row House

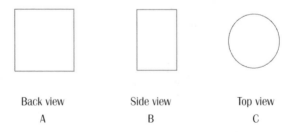

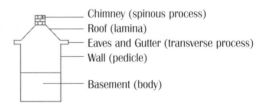

Figure 1 - 6

"Blueprint" Views of a Vertebral Body

| Back view | Side view | Top view |
| A | B | C |

The main part of the vertebra, called the **body**, is a thick cylinder of bone—the basement of our row house. In the neck, the cylinder is shorter and smaller in diameter than it is in the lumbar spine, where the cylinder is about 1 inch (2.5 centimeters) high and 1.2 inches (3 centimeters) in diameter. (**Fig. 1–7A**) The outer surface of the body is a dense, hard type of bone called the **cortex**. The inside is spongy marrow. The cylinder is oriented up and down—like an oil drum placed end-up on the ground. (**Fig. 1–7B**) The body of the vertebra is the front part of the vertebra. It's closest to the face in the neck region and to the abdominal cavity in the lumbar region.

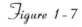

Figure 1 - 7

Vertebral Body and Oil Drum

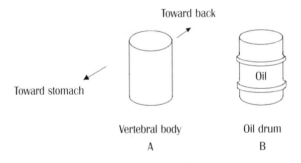

Toward back

Toward stomach

Oil

Vertebral body
A

Oil drum
B

Just as walls rise up above the basement of a row house, so do walls or pillars rise from the round, cylindrical part of the vertebral body. These pillars, or **pedicles**, are mostly dense bone and are quite rigid. (**Fig.1– 8**) There is a space between the pillars of one vertebra and the pillars of the next. This space, as you will see later, is the opening through which the spinal nerves come.

Figure 1-8

"Blueprint" Views of the Vertebral Pedicles

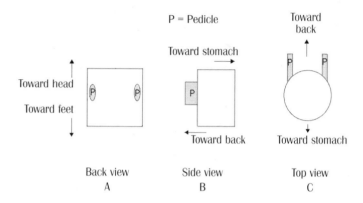

Back view
A

Side view
B

Top view
C

A house without a roof is useless and won't provide much protection for the people living inside. So, too, the pedicles of the vertebra are connected by a roof. (**Fig. 1–9**)

Figure 1-9

"Blueprint" Views of the Vertebral Laminae

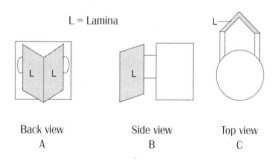

Back view
A

Side view
B

Top view
C

Latin Lesson

Each half of the roof of a vertebra is called a **lamina**, again a feminine Latin noun. There are two half roofs, which are solidly fused to their respective pedicles and to each other in the middle. The two together are called **laminae**.

The vertebra even has a structure that mimics a chimney at the top of the roof; it is called a **spinous process** and serves as the point of attachment of a special gristle tissue. (**Fig. 1–10**)

Figure 1 - 10

"Blueprint" Views of Vertebral Spinous Process

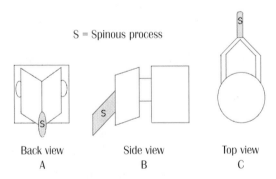

S = Spinous process

Back view
A

Side view
B

Top view
C

It's the part of the spine you feel every time you run your fingers up and down your significant other's back. The tip of the spinous process is, in a normal adult, about 0.5 inch (1.2 centimeters) below the surface of the skin of the back. Sticking out horizontally from each lamina (or roof half) where it attaches to the pedicle is another bony projection called a **transverse process**—like the rain gutter running along a roof edge. (**Fig. 1–11**) In the midback, or thoracic spine, the transverse processes are the structures to which the ribs attach. But in the neck and lumbar spine, there are no ribs, so the transverse processes have nothing to do.

Figure 1 - 11

"Blueprint" Views of Vertebral Transverse Processes

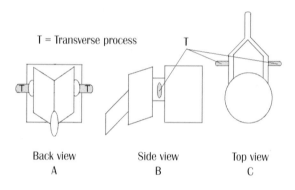

T = Transverse process

| Back view | Side view | Top view |
| A | B | C |

Now I've described the houses, the twenty-four individual vertebrae of the neck, midback, and low back. But they aren't really row houses yet because they haven't been connected to each other. A number of specialized structures do this job, and each of them, as you will see later on, can be the cause of back or neck pain. None of these specialized structures is made of bone; instead, they are all made of different types of gristle tissue and are collectively called **soft tissues**.

The Intervertebral Disc

The first and, in many ways, most important of these structures is the **intervertebral disc**, which is simply called "the disc."

ℱigure 1 - 12

"Blueprint" Drawing of an Intervertebral Disc

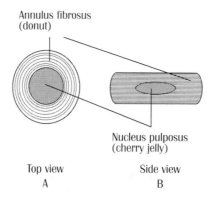

Annulus fibrosus
(donut)

Nucleus pulposus
(cherry jelly)

Top view   Side view
A   B

The disc fits between and is tightly connected to the flat, round ends of the bodies of two adjacent vertebrae and is the same diameter as they are. Discs vary in height, however, from less than 0.25 inch (0.7 centimeter) thick in the neck (cervical region) to almost 0.75 inch (2 centimeters) thick in the low back (lumbar region). Discs are 80 percent water, with most of the water being contained within the nucleus pulposus (the cherry jelly). They eliminate what would be a terrible jarring every time you take a step and your foot hits the ground. They also allow the spine to bend forward and sideward, straighten, and twist. (**Fig. 1–13**)

Figure 1 - 13

"Blueprint" Views of Discs Cushioning Vertebrae

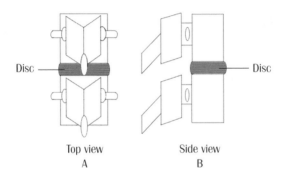

Top view   Side view
A   B

We used to think that discs didn't begin to age and lose any of their water until at least the age of twenty-five. Since the MRI scan came into existence, however, we have learned that discs can age and lose some water in children as young as fifteen or sixteen!

Alphabet Soup: The MRI Scan

MRI stands for "magnetic resonance imaging." It's a computer-generated picture of structures inside the body. You'll learn all about how it's done in chapter 2.

The Spinal Ligaments

The second of the specialized soft tissues that connect the vertebrae together are a group of ligaments. Ligaments are a dense, thick form of gristle tissue that hold two bony structures together. In the spine, ligaments connect each part of one vertebra to the corresponding part of the next. They are all named by their location, and injuries to certain parts of certain ligaments can result in exquisite back pain.

There's a ligament that runs all along the fronts of the bodies of all of the vertebrae. In medicine, *anterior* means "front," so this ligament is called the **anterior longitudinal ligament**. (**Fig. 1–14**)

Figure 1 - 14

"Blueprint" Views of the Anterior Longitudinal Ligament

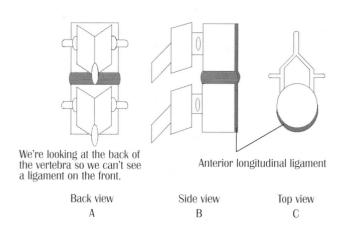

We're looking at the back of the vertebra so we can't see a ligament on the front.

Anterior longitudinal ligament

Back view   Side view   Top view
  A   B   C

The anterior longitudinal ligament has a sibling that runs along the backs of the bodies of all of the vertebrae. In medicine, *posterior* means "back," so this ligament is called the **posterior longitudinal ligament**. It is of particular importance because it also covers the posterior, or back, portion of each disc and helps hold the disc in place. (**Fig. 1–15**) You'll hear a lot more about this when I discuss ruptured discs.

Figure 1 - 15

"Blueprint" Views of the Posterior Longitudinal Ligament

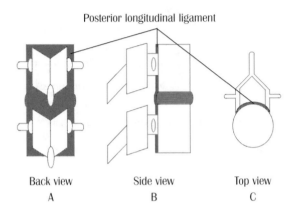

Posterior longitudinal ligament

Back view	Side view	Top view
A	B	C

There's also a ligament that connects each spinous process (the chimney on top of the roof) to the next. This is called the **interspinous ligament**. **(Fig. 1–16)**

Figure 1 - 16

"Blueprint" Views of the Interspinous Ligament

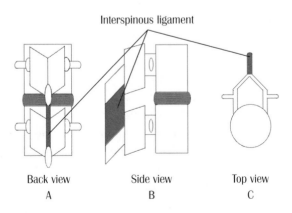

Interspinous ligament

Back view	Side view	Top view
A	B	C

A different ligament connects each transverse process (the rain gutter) to the next: the **intertransverse ligament**. (**Fig. 1–17**)

Figure 1 - 17

"Blueprint" Views of the Intertransverse Ligament

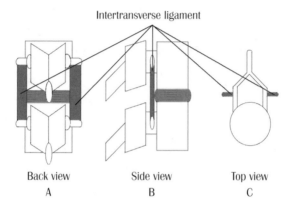

Intertransverse ligament

Back view	Side view	Top view
A	B	C

Finally, there's a ligament that connects each half of the roof—the lamina—to the next. You'd think that, from the way we're going, it would be called the interlaminar ligament, right? Wrong! It's really called the **ligamentum flavum**. (**Fig. 1–18**)

Quick History Lesson

When someone struck a match and lit a candle, thus ending the Dark Ages, learning began to flourish in Europe. Universities sprang up all over Italy and attracted thousands of people, many of whom came to watch anatomists dissect cadavers. (Never say those Renaissance folk didn't know how to have fun.)

As they learned about the insides of the human body, they gave names to the structures they found. When they dissected the spine, they saw the ligament connecting one lamina to the next, and noted that it was intensely yellow. So they said, "Wow! Look at that yellow ligament!" But they were speaking Latin, the language of learning, and so they actually said, "*Ecce! Ligamentum flavum!*" Ever since, it's been called the *ligamentum flavum*. (Yep, *flavum* means "yellow.")

Figure 1 - 18

"Blueprint" Views of the Ligamentum Flavum

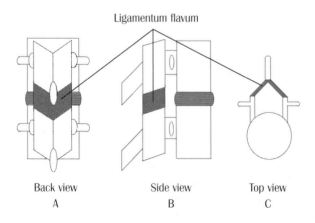

Ligamentum flavum

Back view	Side view	Top view
A	B	C

The Paraspinal Muscles

The final set of specialized soft tissues that connect the vertebrae are the muscles. Basically, there's a muscle that goes from a bony area of one vertebra to the corresponding bony areas of many other vertebrae. The muscles attach to the posterior, or back, surfaces of the laminae and the transverse processes, and to the spinous processes. There are many of them—and they all have Latin names—but we medical folk like to make our lives simple, so we simply call them collectively the **paraspinal muscles**. (**Fig. 1–19**)

Figure 1 - 19

"Blueprint" Views of the Paraspinal Muscles

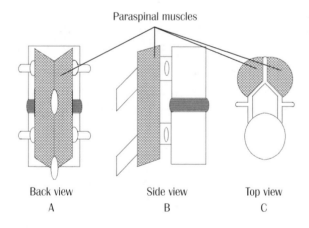

Muscles do only one thing: They contract, or shorten. So when all the muscles on the laminae contract and shorten, they pull you upright and straighten you, a motion we call **extension**. (**Fig. 1–20A**) When the muscles on, say, the right laminae and the right transverse processes contract, they tilt you to the right, a motion we call **side bending**. (**Fig. 1–20B**)

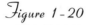

Figure 1 - 20

Muscle Movement

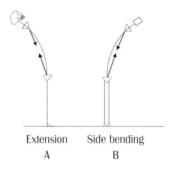

Extension	Side bending
A	B

But how do you bend forward—a motion we call **flexion**? All of the paraspinal muscles are on the posterior, or back, side of the vertebrae, and since they can only shorten, there's no way to bend forward. Ah, but there is: The abdominal muscles in the front of your abdomen (also known as the stomach muscles) are responsible for this motion. When they contract, you get pulled forward or bent over—or you flex. (**Fig. 1–21**) Other abdominal muscles off to the sides allow you to twist.

Figure 1 - 21

Forward Flexion

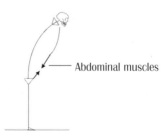

Abdominal muscles

Now that we've learned about the bones, the discs, the ligaments, and the paraspinal muscles, we've begun to get an inkling of how they can be involved in causing pain. But we're not quite ready to dive into that yet. We need to learn about one more very important thing: the inhabitants of our spinal row houses—the spinal cord and the spinal nerve roots.

The Spinal Canal

We all know that the brain is contained within the skull. The bottom of the brain becomes the spinal cord, which leaves the bottom of the skull and travels down through the center of the vertebrae in the **spinal canal**. The floor of the spinal canal is formed by the posterior (back) sides of the bodies of the vertebrae and intervertebral discs—and remember that they are actually covered by the posterior longitudinal ligament.

The sides of the spinal canal are formed by the pedicles—the pillars or walls of the vertebrae. And the roof of the spinal canal is formed by the underside of the laminae (the roof halves) as well as the ligamentum flavum that connects each lamina to the next. (**Fig. 1–22**)

Figure 1-22

The Spinal Canal

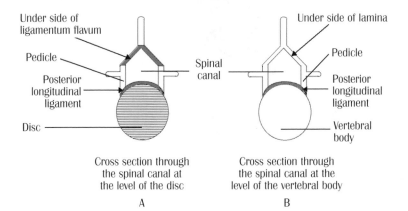

Under side of
ligamentum flavum

Pedicle

Posterior
longitudinal
ligament

Disc

Spinal
canal

Under side of lamina

Pedicle

Posterior
longitudinal
ligament

Vertebral
body

Cross section through
the spinal canal at
the level of the disc

A

Cross section through
the spinal canal at the
level of the vertebral body

B

The pedicles, laminae, and posterior surface of the vertebral bodies and discs (and their covering posterior longitudinal ligament) make a strong, rigid structure and provide good protection for the spinal cord and nerve roots that lie inside and occupy the spinal canal.

Nothing connects one pedicle to the next; there's an open space between them called the *Intervertebral Foramina*, and that's where the individual spinal nerve roots exit as they split off from the spinal cord and go out to the body to supply nerves to all the parts of the body. (**Fig. 1–23**) Between each two vertebrae, on both the right and left sides, a spinal nerve root exits at every level from the neck all the way to the sacrum, the base of the spine. (**Fig. 1–24**)

Figure 1 - 23

Intervertebral Foramina and Nerve Roots

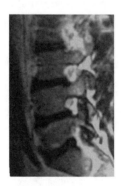

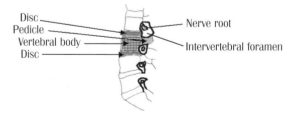

Disc
Pedicle
Vertebral body
Disc

Nerve root
Intervertebral foramen

X-ray Vision

This MRI scan on page 20 is a slice that is about 1 centimeter away from the center line of the vertebra:

Plane of MRI slice ⎯⎯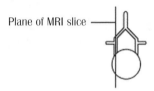

As a result, this slice goes through the pedicle and shows how the pedicle extends back from the vertebral body. You cannot see the spinous process on this slice because the spinous process is in the center line, called the **midline**.

Figure 1 - 24

"Blueprint" Views of the Spinal Nerve Roots

S = Spinal nerve roots   E = Exiting nerve root

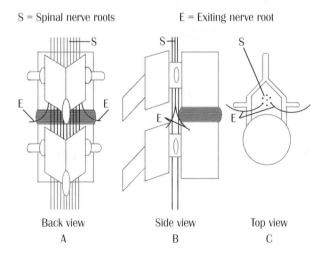

Back view   Side view   Top view
A   B   C

Interestingly, the spinal cord itself actually ends between the first and second lumbar vertebrae, at the upper end of the low back region. (We count vertebrae from the head downward.) After that, the spinal nerve roots continue on down the spinal canal by themselves, a pair continuing to exit right and left between each two vertebrae. As those lower lumbar and sacral spinal nerves descend through the spinal canal, they look like the tail of a horse, and that's exactly what they're called—in Latin, of course—the **cauda equina**. (**Fig. 1–25**)

Figure 1 - 25

Cauda Equina

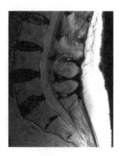

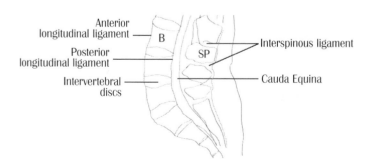

X-ray Vision

The MRI scan on page 22 is a slice that goes through the midline of the vertebra.

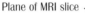 Plane of MRI slice

This slice goes through the spinous process **(SP)** so the pedicle, being a centimeter away from the midline, is not seen. You can see the anterior longitudinal ligament, the posterior longitudinal ligament, the interspinous ligament, the intervertebral discs, and the vertebral bodies **(B)**.

Now that you've learned about all the structures that make up the spine, it will be easy for you to understand how they can be injured, the kinds of pain those injuries can cause, the ways we diagnose those pains, and how we can treat them.

Chapter Two

History Lessons
The Key to a Successful Diagnosis

It's almost like a magic trick: You go to the doctor, and before you even finish describing your problem, the doctor nods sagely and pronounces your diagnosis. In fact, some doctors might even relish your awe at their ability to (seemingly) pluck the correct diagnosis out of thin air. But medicine isn't magic; diagnoses are made by following a highly ritualized process of thinking and doing in a very ordered and logical manner.

Almost all doctors, for example, organize their office notes in a form called **SOAP**, which is an acronym for **subjective, objective, assessment**, and **plan**.

Subjective	The patient's own perception of what seems to be wrong
Objective	The doctor's examination of the patient, based on the patient's description of complaints
Assessment	The doctor's decision on how the examination relates to the symptoms and what diagnosis (or diagnoses) can be attached to that combination
Plan	The treatment the doctor prescribes for the diagnosis that's been made

This logical format carries over into the actual way the office visit is conducted.

At the Doctor's Office

When you meet the doctor, you're first asked for a **history**. The history is simply a chronologic story of everything that's happened from the moment you injured your back until the moment the doctor first sees you. It begins with the **chief complaint**: your reason for having come to the doctor. The chief complaint may be, "I bent over to pick up a paper on the floor, and I got a sudden, sharp pain in my low back," or, "I played in a pickup basketball game two days ago, and now my neck is sore," or, "I woke up this morning, and my back is stiff, and I don't know why."

The doctor will then ask you questions to try to figure out what happened and how it happened. You'll be asked whether the pain came on immediately or gradually, whether it's sharp or dull, whether it stays in one place or radiates from the back to the leg, whether it's constant or intermittent, if there's any numbness or tingling, and so forth. Don't be irritated by all the questions—your doctor needs this information to determine where the pain arose and what structure or structures might be responsible for it. In fact, in orthopaedics, we say that 85 percent of the time we can make a diagnosis purely on the basis of a thorough history!

The Physical Examination

After taking the history, the doctor will perform a **physical examination**. The orthopaedic exams of the neck and the low back both follow the same basic format:

✦ **Inspection.** This merely means looking at the area. You'd be surprised what a doctor can pick up just by observing the low back. Remember that C-shaped curve I discussed in chapter 1, where the midpart of the C faces toward the front as a patient is viewed from the side? (**Fig. 2–1A**) Well, an absence of lordosis can be a sign of muscle spasm. (**Fig. 2–1B**) In the low back, a shift off to the right or left—a condition called a **sciatic shift**—is also a sign of intense muscle spasm. (**Fig. 2–1C**) The doctor's trained eye can pick up many other visible signs that help determine a diagnosis.

Figure 2-1

Physical Examination: What Can Be Seen on Inspection

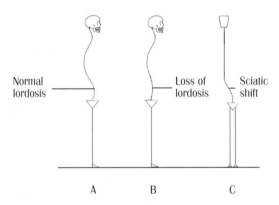

Normal lordosis   Loss of lordosis   Sciatic shift

A   B   C

◆ **Palpation.** This is just a fancy medical term for poking around. Your doctor palpates by using his fingertips to feel all over the area being inspected. Contrary to what you might think, he's not trying to annoy you—he's actually looking for two more clues: areas of tenderness and areas of spasm. Tenderness might be present over a bone, a muscle, or a ligament—or a combination of them. Spasm will be found over muscles. Spasm is, unfortunately, frequently overdiagnosed; ideally, it should be accompanied by a loss of lordosis. In rare instances, palpation can reveal an area of intense heat, which could indicate the possibility of infection deep in the tissues below that region.

Another part of palpation is **percussion**, which means tapping. Your doctor can tap (or less euphemistically, hit) along the spinous processes of the vertebrae, the interspinous ligament that connects them, or the paraspinal muscles. Pain on percussion can have specific diagnostic significance in certain cases.

✦ **Range of motion.** Here, the doctor asks you to bend forward
(flex), bend backward (extend), bend to the right and left,
and rotate or twist to the right and left. This part of the
exam is, of course, accompanied by both inspection and
palpation. If there is limitation of motion, your doctor can
easily see whether or not it is accompanied by pain or spasm. If
your back is normal, when you bend forward the lumbar lordotic curve reverses, and you have a nice kyphotic curve, or
kyphosis, from the thoracic spine all the way to the sacrum
(the tailbone). (**Fig. 2–2A**) If there's spasm, however, the
lumbar lordotic curve will not reverse, and the lumbar area
will look flat. (**Fig. 2–2B**) In the low back, doctors can also see
something called segmental spasm. The normal lumbar spine
makes a smooth C-shaped curve when it bends to the right or
left, (**Fig. 2–3A**) but if muscle spasm is present, frequently the
low back will look as if it consists of two straight lines that
bend at only one spot. (**Fig. 2–3B**)

ℑigure 2-2

Physical Examination: What Can be Seen During Range of Motion

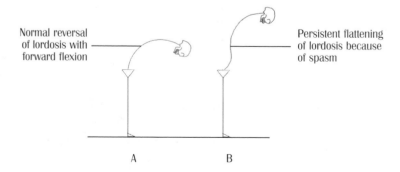

Normal reversal
of lordosis with
forward flexion

Persistent flattening
of lordosis because
of spasm

A   B

Figure 2-3

Physical Examination: What Can be Seen During Range of Motion

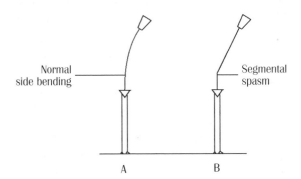

Normal side bending — | Segmental spasm

A   B

✦ **A series of orthopaedic and neurologic tests.** These tests assess the status of the bones, joints, muscles, tendons, ligaments, nerves, arteries, and veins of the arms or legs. Why check your legs if your low back aches? Because the spinal nerves that supply the legs originate in the low back. Your doctor needs to know if irritation or pressure on those nerves is part of the reason for your back pain. Even though the doctor can't see the nerves in the spinal canal in the low back, he can check the things that those spinal nerves control in the legs and infer which nerve is causing the problem.

The orthopaedic tests. This consists again of inspection and palpation of the entire length of both legs, and examines a range of motion of all the joints from from the hips to the toes. In addition, a manual muscle exam is performed. Each individual major muscle from the hips to the toes can be specifically tested to determine its strength. Remember, I said in chapter 1 that muscles do only one thing: They contract, or shorten. All muscles should have a grade of normal, meaning that they should be able to contract, or shorten, through a full range of motion against both gravity and resistance. If a certain muscle—or a group of muscles all supplied by the same spinal nerve—is weaker than normal, that immediately indicates which spinal nerve is irritated. The doctor should also test for the integrity of the ligaments that span each joint and of the lining of each of the joints (remember that ligaments are a dense, thick form of gristle tissue that hold two bony structures together).

A quick form of the manual muscle exam is to have the patient walk on his toes and heels. If the patient can toe walk, the muscles on the back of the calf have enough strength to raise the body against the force of its own weight and against the force of gravity and simultaneously propel the body forward. If the patient can heel walk, the muscles on the front of the calf have enough strength to raise the foot and toes against the force of gravity and simultaneously propel the body forward. Muscles that can do these things have a grade of normal.

The neurologic tests. This includes testing for reflexes and sensation. Almost everyone has seen a doctor tap just below the knee with a little reflex hammer and then watch the lower leg jump. That's the knee-jerk reflex. The doctor is actually tapping on the tendon that connects the lower end of the kneecap (called the patella) to the upper part of the shinbone (the tibia). When that tendon is tapped, a signal goes from a special nerve ending in that tendon to the spinal cord and then down to the muscle on the front of the thigh, making it contract and pull up (straightening) the lower leg below the knee. Reflexes are graded with a number from 0 (nothing at all happens) to 4+ (a condition called hyperreflexia), along with an indication of whether the reflex occurs briskly or sluggishly. A normal reflex is described as "2+ and brisk." In addition to the knee-jerk reflex (or patellar tendon reflex), in the leg, there's a reflex behind the ankle involving the Achilles tendon called the ankle-jerk reflex or the Achilles reflex (which can also be called by its medical term, the gastro-soleus tendon reflex). When a doctor tests for sensation, he tests for pinprick as well as light touch (sharp and dull), felt by two different types of nerve endings. You'll learn more about this later.

Here's an important anatomic fact that isn't generally known by laypeople: The special parts of the nerves that come from the spinal cord and supply sensation to the arms and legs do so in longitudinal bands called **dermatomes**. **(Fig. 2-4)**

Figure 2-4

The Dermatomes of the Leg

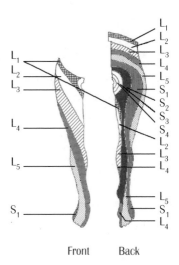

L = the dermotome supplied by a lumbar nerve root. L_1, for example, is the dermatome supplied by the first lumbar nerve root. S_1 is supplied by the first sacral nerve root.

Front   Back

Testing, Testing

As I said earlier, in orthopaedics, a diagnosis can be made 85 percent of the time just on the basis of the history. The physical examination increases a doctor's ability to make a diagnosis to 95 percent. So what can a doctor do to make a diagnosis in that remaining 5 percent of cases when the history and physical exam haven't provided enough information?

The answer may lie in the results of **diagnostic tests** that can be performed. There are a number of such tests that the doctor can order, and they range from simple to quite complex.

X-RAY

X-rays are the first tests ordered by the doctor to see exactly how the bones of the back appear. In fact, that's all x-rays do: They show bones because almost the only things that show up on an x-ray are structures that contain calcium. They don't show muscles, ligaments, tendons, nerves, discs, arteries, or veins. Sometimes certain shadows will occur as a result of air in tissues like the throat or because of a difference in density between areas of fat and of muscle. Those shadows can be helpful in pointing toward a diagnosis. X-rays can't show a sprain or strain or any soft-tissue injury (an injury to muscles, tendons, or ligaments). They *can* show arthritis, a fracture, a tumor in the bone, or an infection. A regular (or **plane**) x-ray is merely a flat, two-dimensional longitudinal picture of a part of the body. This means that, for example, a front- or side-view x-ray of the spine will look like the picture of a skeleton. (**Fig. 2–5**)

CAT SCAN

CAT stands for "computerized axial tomography." A CAT scan is a very fancy x-ray study in which a computer-controlled x-ray machine takes a whole lot of x-rays from inside what looks like a giant dough-nut. The patient lies on a special x-ray table that is slid into the hole of the doughnut. If you think of the doughnut as a clock, x-rays are taken while the computer aims from every hour. The computer soft-ware then takes all the x-ray pictures that were made "around the clock" and turns them into slices through a part of the body. Think of a loaf of sliced bread. If the whole loaf represented, say, four or five vertebrae, then each slice would represent a picture *across* part of one vertebra—a cross section. The CAT scan can show bones, discs, and muscles very well. It can show—with less detail—arteries, veins, and nerves. (**Fig. 2–6**) It's good for showing a herniated disc, arthritis, tu-mor, and infection.

Figure 2-5

Normal Lumbar Spine

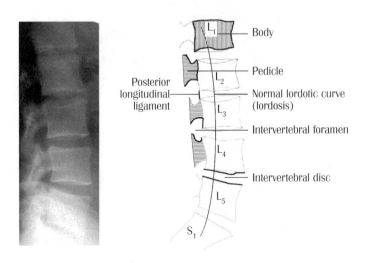

X-ray Vision

The x-ray on page 33 is a side view, or lateral, x-ray of the lumbar spine. Notice that all of the vertebral bodies are square and that all the spaces for the intervertebral discs are the same height. Remember that the posterior longitudinal ligament, which runs along the back (or posterior) surface of the vertebral bodies and the discs, is invisible on an x-ray. You can see on the illustration where it is actually located.

Figure 2-6

CAT Scan Cross Section

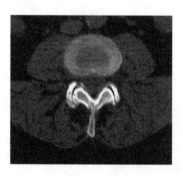

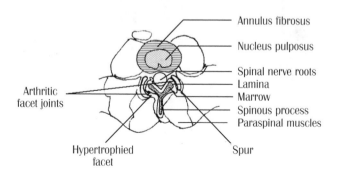

Annulus fibrosus
Nucleus pulposus
Spinal nerve roots
Lamina
Marrow
Spinous process
Paraspinal muscles

Arthritic facet joints

Hypertrophied facet

Spur

X-ray Vision

We can see the normal nucleus pulposus separate from the annulus fibrosus of the intervertebral disc on the CAT scan on page 34. We see a normal spinal canal with the spinal nerve roots taking up most of its space. Although the disc, spinal canal, and nerve roots are all normal, the bones are not. We see arthritic facet joints, which are narrowed. The facet has hypertrophied and formed a large spur which has markedly distorted its normal appearance. There is a smaller spur, that has started to form on the other side.

MRI SCAN

MRI stands for magnetic resonance imaging. An MRI scan is *not* an x-ray. You'll need to review a little physics in order to understand how it's done and what it is. I promise I'll make it simple! The MRI scan is based on the fact that all the tissues of the body contain water. In fact, the body is 80 percent water. There's water in bones, muscles, ligaments, nerves, and, of course, blood vessels. Water is a molecule composed of two hydrogen atoms and one oxygen atom—the world-famous H_2O. Each atom has tiny electrical particles within it. These electrical particles can be caused to move to a different (or higher) energy state if a very strong magnetic field is brought near them. When the strong magnetic field is taken away, they then go back to their original energy state. What makes this so fascinating—and what makes the MRI scan such an excellent tool—is that the *speed* at which energy states change varies with each type of tissue in the presence of a strong magnetic field. In other words, the rate of change for the energy state of the electrical particles of water molecules of bone is different from that of muscle . . . which is different still from that of ligaments . . . and of nerves, and so on.

An MRI scanner is a long cylinder that is a giant permanent magnet. The best ones currently in use create a magnetic field that is *sixty thousand* times the background magnetic field found on the earth. The patient lies on a narrow table that slides into the long cylinder. The intense magnetic field generated by the permanent magnet causes all the electrical charges of the water atoms to line up the same way. Then a computer rapidly turns on and off an electromagnet inside the long cylinder. Every time the electromagnet is turned on, the electrical charges jump to a new energy state; when the electromagnet is turned off, they go back to their original energy state. But remember that they do this at different speeds, and the computer can sense *exactly where every collection of atoms changing at each speed is located.*

The computer prints out a "map" of where all of them are located, and this map is actually a picture of a part of the body. Remember, I said that the CAT scan only shows cross sections (like a slice of bread). The MRI scan can show not only cross sections, (**Fig. 2–7**) but also longitudinal sections—picture a loaf of bread that's been sliced from top to bottom lengthwise—and coronal sections, which resemble a hot-dog roll that's been sliced.

Figure 2-7

MRI Scan Cross Section

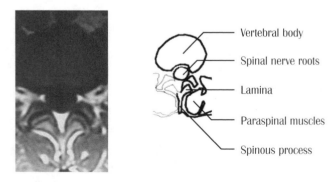

Vertebral body

Spinal nerve roots

Lamina

Paraspinal muscles

Spinous process

X-Ray Vision

I've rotated the MRI picture on page 36 so that it's oriented the same as the "Blueprint" drawings in Chapter 1. Normally, MRI cross sections are oriented with the spinous process pointing down, and that will be the way others are shown. It looks like there's no room between the spinal nerve roots and the lamina, but there really is. We already saw a longitudinal MRI scan section in Figure 1-23.

MRI scanners with big magnets and updated computer software can make pictures that show bones, muscles, ligaments, tendons, nerves (including spinal nerves), discs, and blood vessels, all with excellent detail. These pictures can show incredibly helpful detail, such as when discs have lost some of their water (from the "cherry jelly" or nucleus pulposus) and have degenerated, hemorrhage in muscles that have been torn, swelling of nerves, and more. The MRI scan thus shows a herniated disc, arthritis, infection, and tumor. Sometimes a dye called gadolinium is injected into an arm vein midway through an MRI scan. This provides greater contrast between normal and abnormal tissues on the MRI pictures.

BONE SCAN

This is a test in which a minute quantity of radioactive dye is injected into a vein. The dye then circulates throughout the body and eventually settles in bones. (It doesn't take long for the body to get rid of the dye; almost all of it is gone in less than twenty-four hours.) When the bone scan is performed, the patient lies on a special table. As the dye is injected, a fancy Geiger counter called a gamma camera scans the body and sees how the dye flows, giving a general idea of the state of the circulatory system, the first phase. A computer creates a picture of this. Additional pictures are taken after several minutes, showing if the dye has pooled

in any area(s), the way it would if extra blood vessels had formed—
an indication of a possible infection or tumor, the second phase.

The patient is then allowed to get up and walk around and comes
back three hours later for a final set of pictures that show if the dye has
concentrated in one or more areas of bone, the third phase. (**Fig. 2–8**)
The bone scan shows evidence of conditions such as arthritis, fracture,
infection, tumor, and more. It does not show actual bones or soft tissues.

Figure 2-8

Bone Scan

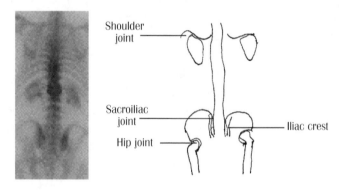

X-ray Vision

This is a scan taken three hours after the dye was injected. The dye
has equilibrated and is evenly distributed throughout the bony skeleton. There are no signs of arthritis in the hip joints or the shoulder
joints. The sacroiliac joints are not arthritic; the dark area there represents increased dye in the marrow of the iliac crest.

MYELOGRAM

A myelogram is an x-ray test that's used because the spinal cord, spinal nerve roots, and intervertebral disc are all invisible on a plane x-ray. When a myelogram is performed, a long needle is inserted through the skin of the back (what, you don't think that sounds like fun?) and then advanced through successive layers: fatty tissue, the gristle covering the paraspinal muscles, the paraspinal muscles themselves, the ligamentum flavum (remember the "yellow ligament"?), and into the spinal canal. The needle then is carefully pushed through the covering of the spinal cord (called the **dura or thecal sac**). Iodine dye is injected inside the dura and flows between it and the spinal cord. X-rays are taken with the patient in different positions. Arthritis or a herniated disc will push against the column of dye and indent it, and that indentation can be seen on the x-rays. (**Fig. 2–9**)

Figure 2-9

Lumbar Myelogram

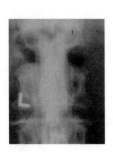 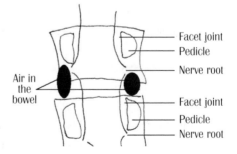

X-ray Vision

The facet joints and pedicles are not enlarged or arthritic, so the column of dye flows straight with no indentations. Notice how the spinal nerve roots exit just below the pedicles on this front view x-ray. Those dark circles are air in the bowel. Remember this is a two-dimensional picture, so the overlying abdominal cavity and its contents are superimposed on the spine and thecal sac.

DISCOGRAM

A discogram is an x-ray test that's similar to the myelogram, but with one big difference: When the long needle is inserted through all the layers, it comes in farther from the side, away from the ligamentum flavum. It is then aimed into the disc and completely avoids the dura. The theory is that the needle ends up in the center of the cherry jelly—the nucleus pulposus. The same dye that's used in the myelogram is used in the discogram and is then injected into the nucleus pulposus. (Remember, the disc is otherwise invisible on an x-ray.) After the dye is injected, x-rays are taken from the front and from the side. If the dye remains within the nucleus pulposus, it means the disc is normal. If the dye leaks out into the annulus fibrosus (the thick gristle ring or doughnut), the disc is degenerated. If the dye flows out from the annulus fibrosus, through the posterior longitudinal ligament (the ligament that runs along the back surfaces of the discs and the bodies of the vertebrae), the disc is herniated. (**Fig. 2–10**)

It's a great theory, and when it works right it's terrific. The problem is that the needle has to be *centered* in the nucleus pulposus. If it's just a little off to the side (above, below, behind, in front of, to the right, or to the left of the cherry jelly) and is actually in the annulus fibrosus, the discogram is invalid. The reason is that dye in the annulus fibrosus is automatically considered to represent a degenerated disc, and if the needle is in the annulus rather than the nucleus, that's where the dye will be injected, rather than having the dye leak out from a degenerated nucleus into the annulus. Perfect front and side x-rays are necessary to see where the needle is placed, and the margin of error is only a few millimeters.

Figure 2-10

Discogram

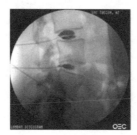

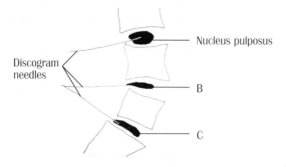

Nucleus pulposus

Discogram needles

B

C

X-ray Vision

In this discogram, all three needles have been placed in the centers of the three nuclei pulposi (the cherry jelly). The uppermost of the three discs is normal, with all of the dye contained inside the nucleus pulposus. The middle disc is markedly abnormal. Notice how dye has leaked out of the disc and into the annulus fibrosus **(B)**, and has even leaked into the spinal canal **(C)**.

Another problem is that a healthy disc will admit only a very small amount of dye. A degenerated disc will accept more dye. When the dye is injected, if the patient has sudden pain, that's taken to mean that the disc is not only degenerated but is also the cause of the patient's symptoms. Of course, if the needle is in the annulus to begin with, then dye being injected into it may cause pain even if the disc is not the source of the problem. Many people cite a false positive rate of up to 60 percent for discograms. This means that up to 60 percent may look as if they are positive for a herniated, degenerative, or symptomatic disc when, in fact, the discs are okay. Most other studies—electrocardiograms, blood tests, and other x-ray studies for example—have false positive rates of well under 5 percent, with some even well under 1 percent.

ELECTROMYOGRAMS AND NERVE CONDUCTION TESTS

EMGs and NCTs, as we medical cognocenti call them, test the ability of nerves to transmit signals and the ability of muscles to receive those signals. Doctors can't go sticking needles into the spinal cord or the spinal nerve roots that branch off from it inside the spinal canal. But we know that each spinal nerve root has a particular muscle or muscles that it supplies. (You learned earlier in this chapter that each spinal nerve root also supplies a specific area of skin with feeling or sensation.)

It *is* possible to stick a very thin needle electrode into a muscle, test how it is functioning, and thus infer how the nerve root that supplies that muscle is functioning. That's what an EMG does. The electromyographer inserts the needle electrode into a muscle while looking at an oscilloscope to which the electrode is connected. He observes an "insertional pattern" on the oscilloscope. Then the patient keeps still, and the "resting pattern" is seen. Next, the patient makes the muscle twitch a little, and a "minimal contraction pattern" occurs. The patient then tightens the muscle, and a "maximum contraction pattern" is seen. Ideally, five separate areas of each muscle should be sampled, which means that the patient sort of becomes a pincushion. (Kind of makes that single-needle test sound good, doesn't it?)

The NCT, as the name indicates, tests the ability of a nerve to conduct impulses. Several spinal nerve roots join together to make a nerve trunk. This trunk includes both sensory fibers that supply sensation (hot, cold, touch, pressure, and so on), and motor fibers (fibers that make muscles contract). Branches containing both motor and sensory fibers split off from the trunk and become the nerves that go to a particular part of the body. Some of those nerves are fairly close to the skin. The electromyographer places two electrode pads (similar to those used when you have a cardiogram performed) a measured distance apart over the nerve. An electrical impulse is sent to one electrode. It then stimulates the nerve, which conducts the impulse along its course. The second electrode senses when that nerve impulse passes it, and a machine measures the time (in milliseconds) it takes to get from one electrode to the next—the nerve conduction time. The electromyographer can determine how long it takes for the nerve to realize it's been stimulated (the latency), the quality of the conducted impulse (the amplitude), the duration of the conducted impulse, and more. This information can tell us if the nerve is "pinched" (impinged upon by disc pressure or spinal arthritis).

Now that you've earned your Junior Doctor's Merit Badge, it's time to take all the information I've given you on the structure and function of the spine and on how doctors try to diagnose what's wrong and put it to good use!

Chapter Three

GETTING TO THE HEART
OF YOUR BACK PAIN
HOW THE BACK GETS HURT

In this chapter, I'll discuss acute injuries and problems—the kind of back pain that comes on suddenly after a specific incident. (In the next chapter, you'll learn about chronic conditions—those that slowly develop over a period of years and that may, from time to time, suddenly become painful.) Moving on to acute pain. For example, you might have bent over to pick up a carton of books, tried to open a stuck window, lifted or carried a heavy load of laundry, played tennis and lunged to make a return, or you might have been involved in a motor vehicle accident. Perhaps you slipped and fell on an icy sidewalk. Maybe all you did was roll around on the floor while playing with your kids.

All of these activities can cause lower back pain. In fact, they can cause the *same kinds* of symptoms. The symptoms can actually be identical in each of these injuries—and yet each of these injuries may be entirely different!

The injury may be a **sprain** or **strain**, an irritation of a specialized joint in the back, a ligament injury, a stretch or irritation of a nerve root, a flare-up of arthritis, a fracture or broken bone, or a herniated disc. So how do we figure out what's wrong? Well, putting to use the knowledge just acquired when you earned your Junior Doctor's Merit Badge in chapter 2, we begin with a history. Unfortunately, many of those activities mentioned above can result in a very similar history: They may all have caused the sudden onset of lower back pain, which may—or may not—have radiated down one or both legs, and which may—or may not—have been accompanied by numbness and/or tingling. (The fancy medical word for tingling or pins and needles is **paresthesias**.) But there are often subtle differences in the histories, and that's what I'll concentrate on now.

Junior Doctor's Merit Badge Checkpoint

SPRAIN OR STRAIN: WHAT'S THE DIFFERENCE?

A **sprain** is an injury to a ligament. (Ligaments act like hinges and connect one bone to another.)

A **strain** is an injury to a muscle.

In the neck and low back, the muscles and ligaments are so intimately connected to each other that we can use either *sprain* or *strain* for both, since both are usually injured.

For instance, often the lower back pain associated with a sprain or strain doesn't begin at the moment of injury. Instead, the pain can come on gradually, beginning as early as just an hour or two after the injury, or as long as one to three days afterward. On the other hand, lower back pain associated with a flare-up of arthritis, an irritation of one of the specialized joints in the low back, or with a fracture will usually come on immediately.

In addition, the physical examination helps distinguish among various diagnoses. The numbness and paresthesias that may accompany a back sprain won't result in actual changes that can be observed in tests for sensation or result in diminution of reflexes, while those same symptoms will show change when performed on a patient with a herniated disc.

Let's look at each kind of injury and try to pull all these things together so we can understand how they occur and what they look and
feel like.

Low Back Sprains and Strains

The most common injury to the low back, or lumbar spine, is a sprain
or strain. This can happen as a result of virtually any type of activity:
bending, lifting, carrying, twisting, being involved in sports activities,
and much more. The pain of a sprain/strain, as I just noted, may not
come on immediately—although it certainly can—but may rather arise
gradually over a period of hours or even over several days. The pain is
intense, but frequently it is intermittent, arising only with certain
movements and frequently subsiding with rest. (By *rest*, I mean lying
down.) The pain may radiate rarely into one or both legs; even more
rarely, there may be a feeling of poorly localized numbness or paresthesias. Poorly localized means there's a kind of tingly or numb feeling in
part of one or both legs, but you can't pin down exactly where. As
you'll see later, that's very different from numbness or parasthesias
caused by nerve root irritation.

When a sprain/strain occurs, what actually happens is that the paraspinal muscles and/or ligaments (especially the interspinous and intertransverse ligaments) are suddenly stretched. *Stretched* here doesn't
mean like pulling a rubber band or a piece of taffy. Instead, it refers to a
microscopic distance, literally less than a millimeter. But to the body,
a structure that doesn't stretch at all in normal use will seem to have
stretched the length of a football field when a sudden abnormal motion occurs.

When this happens, individual muscle cells may tear and leak out
their intercellular contents. Tiny capillaries that bring blood to these
muscle cells may also tear, spilling out individual blood cells. Now,
what I'm describing can only be seen under a microscope; I'm not
talking about the kind of bleeding that's visible to the naked eye, such

as you see when you cut your finger. When the contents of individual torn muscle cells and individual red blood cells leak out, they irritate other intact muscle cells. These intact cells react by contracting; in fact, they do so by the thousands and remain almost continuously contracted. This intense contraction is what a patient feels as spasm.

Here's a simplified chart for a patient who is suffering from spasm:

Physical Examination

Inspection

Will show loss of lordosis (poker spine) or a sciatic shift where it looks as if the patient is shifted off to the right or left as we look at the patient from behind. (You can see how this looks in chapter 2, figure 2–1.)

Palpation

Spasm can often be felt as a rigid hardness; the back may be diffusely tender over the paraspinal muscles.

Range of Motion

We may find limitation of motion—often because of pain—but we also may be able to see segmental spasm when the patient bends to the right or left. (The back looks as if it is composed of two straight lines that bend at only one spot rather than a smooth, C-shaped curve.) We may also see persistence of lordosis when the patient bends forward. Normally, when you bend forward or flex, the lumbar lordotic curve reverses and becomes kyphotic: The forward-facing C becomes a backward-facing Ɔ. (You can see how these conditions look in chapter 2, figures 2–2 and 2–3.)

	Persistence of lordosis on forward flexion is an excellent confirmation of spasm because it can't be faked.
Orthopaedic and Neurologic Tests	Will all be normal: Sensation, motor power, reflexes and tests for nerve root irritation will not show any changes because a sprain/strain does not involve any irritation of the spinal nerve roots in the spinal canal, so the muscles, joints, and skin that they supply won't be affected.

Tests You Might Have	What They Might Show
Lumbar Spine X-rays	Normal—they won't show any abnormalities because we can't see muscles or ligaments on routine x-rays. It's very rare that there is so much spasm that the normal lumbar lordotic curve will not show, even though there may be an absence of lordosis on physical exam.

Ligament Injuries

You've just learned that sprains usually involve the interspinous or intertransverse ligaments, and that they are almost always accompanied by strains of the adjacent paraspinal muscles. And in chapter 1, I showed you the various ligaments that connect one vertebra to another. But I cheated. I didn't show you another group of ligaments that can be injured all by themselves without any accompanying muscle strain. These ligaments are called the **sacroiliac ligaments**. They connect the sacrum—the five fused vertebrae that form the base of the spine just below the five lumbar vertebrae—to the **iliac bones**.

The sacroiliac joints measure about 2.5 to 3 inches (6.5 to 7.5 centimeters) in length and about 1 inch (2.5 centimeters) in thickness from front (anterior) to back (posterior) in normal adults. (**Fig. 3–1**) They have an extremely important function: They transmit *the entire weight of the upper half of the body*—from the fifth lumbar vertebra to the top of the skull—to the legs. These joints are tough and unyielding, because the sacrum is kept lined up with the ilium bone (the big pelvic bone) by very dense, inelastic ligaments. Sometimes, however, some of these very dense, inelastic ligaments may be stretched, allowing a tiny amount of motion between the sacrum and the ilium. This tiny amount of motion creates severe pain, and this pain frequently mimics the pain of nerve root irritation from a herniated disc, because the pain starts at the low back and usually radiates down the leg. When you're standing or walking, the downward force of the weight of the upper half of the body tends to make the sacrum slide downward in relation to the ilium if the ligaments have microscopically stretched. We say that there is a shear force applied.

Figure 3-1

The Pelvis and Sacroiliac Joints

Sacroiliac joints

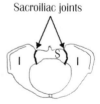

Top view of pelvis

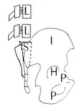

Side view of pelvis

L = Lumbar vertebra
S = Sacrum
I = Ilium (side of pelvis)
P = Pubic bone
(front of pelvis)
H = Hip joint socket

Latin Lesson

The sacrum is actually the back part of the pelvis. On each side of the sacrum is a big, attached hip bone called the ilium or iliac bone. Ilium is Latin, so if we talk about the two of them, the plural is ilia. You can feel the top of each ilium if you run your fingers from your belly button straight around to your side; the top edge is called the iliac crest.

Virtually any of the mechanisms that can cause a sprain/strain of the lumbar spine can also cause a strain of the sacroiliac ligaments. Bending, lifting, and twisting are the most likely causes; sports activities can also result in this problem. The pain associated with this injury usually comes on within a matter of hours. It is intense and often located exactly over the sacroiliac joint. It may disappear when you lie down, but attempting to turn over while lying may cause severe, intense pain. It may be accompanied by pain that radiates down the leg on the side of the irritated sacroiliac joint ligaments (something that's on the same side as something else is called ipsilateral). Usually, but not always, there are no symptoms of numbness or paresthesias. The pain can often be very intense and stabbing, and it may increase with weight bearing. In other words, every time you take a step on the injured side, the pain is worse.

Take a look at the chart for this condition:

PHYSICAL EXAMINATION

Inspection   May show the same findings as for a
                              sprain/strain. Sometimes there may be
                              loss of lordosis or a sciatic shift.

PHYSICAL EXAMINATION

Palpation	This is where we'll learn the most about a ligament injury. Intense pain will be concentrated directly over the irritated sacroiliac joint, not spread out over the lumbar spine.
Range of Motion	Will be limited because of—and accompanied by—intense pain.
Orthopaedic and Neurologic Tests	Normal because, once again, the spinal nerve roots in the spinal canal are not irritated. This is a critical distinction between this injury and a herniated disc (which we'll learn about later).

TESTS YOU MIGHT HAVE | WHAT THEY MIGHT SHOW

Lumbar Spine X-rays	Lumbar spine x-rays (which do include the sacrum and the ilium bones) will look normal because this is a ligament injury. The radiating pain and pseudo-symptoms of numbness and paresthesias that may sometimes occur with this problem may be of such a degree that patients and doctors may be fooled into thinking they are dealing with nerve root irritation.
EMGs and NCTs	Will be normal.
MRI Scan and CAT Scan Studies	Unremarkable.

Note that a careful physical examination should eliminate the need for x-rays, a CAT scan, an MRI scan, or EMGs and NCTs to diagnose most ligament injuries.

Facet Joint Irritation

I have to confess: I cheated again. In chapter 1, I showed you the different parts of a vertebra and described what they do. But I left one out on purpose so I could talk about it now. As you undoubtedly know, when one bone moves in relation to the next, it meets the next at an area called a **joint**. A joint is simply an enclosed space formed by the **apposing** (side by side) ends of two adjacent bones. The tissue that encloses the joint is called the **synovium**. The joints throughout the cervical, thoracic, and lumbar spine function in basically the same way as the shoulder or hip joints: They allow motions in multiple planes.

The bony parts of the joints in the spine are projections that stick out from the pedicles and the laminae.

 Remember: The pedicles are the pillars or walls of our vertebral "houses," and the laminae are the roofs.

The projection from the pedicle faces upward toward the projection coming from the vertebral lamina above it. The projection from the lamina is at its back end and faces downward toward the upward-facing projection from the pedicle below it. Each of these two projections, one sticking out from the pedicle and one sticking out from the lamina, is called a facet. That's because it's a small, fairly flat surface similar to, but larger than, a flat surface or facet on a gemstone.

The facet that projects upward from the pedicle is anterior, and the facet that projects down from the back end of the lamina is posterior. (**Fig. 3–2**)

Figure 3-2

Facet Joints

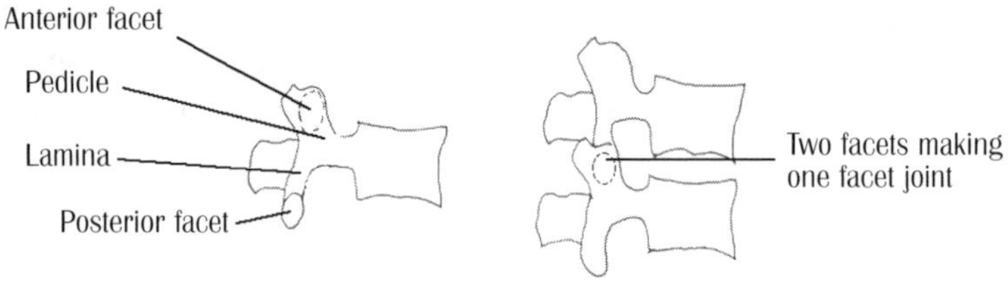

Anterior facet
Pedicle
Lamina
Posterior facet

Two facets making
one facet joint

Side view of vertebrae

Remember: Something toward the front of a bone is called anterior, while something toward the back of a bone is called posterior.

The full name of each is the anterior zygapophyseal facet and the posterior zygapophyseal facet. We can make our lives simple and call each pair of apposing anterior and posterior zygapophyseal facets the *facets*; the two together make one *facet joint*. There's a facet joint on each side of each pair of vertebrae. (**Fig. 3–3A**) They're pretty much lined up like a series of dotted lines such as you see when looking at lane markings on a highway. (**Fig. 3–3B**) When we look at facets end-on, they're angled inward like the top parts of the letter V. (**Fig. 3–4**) It's this unique combination of shapes and alignment that allows the lumbar spine to flex, extend, side bend, and rotate, with each pair of facet joints contributing a small number of degrees toward the total amount of motion.

Figure 3-3

Facet Joint Alignment

F = Facet joint
L = Lamina
S = Spinous process

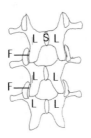

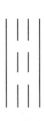

Back view of
vertebrae

A

Dotted lines on
highway

B

Figure 3-4

Plane of Facets Joints

Facets

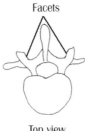

Plane of
facets

Top view

Facet joint irritation is the only acute condition that can be related to an
underlying or preexisting condition. The mechanism for causing a facet

joint injury is the same as for a sprain/strain or sacroiliac ligament injury: bending, twisting, lifting, or the like. Sometimes the pain is localized directly over the injured facet joint; other times, it may be as diffuse as that of a sprain/strain. The pain usually comes on gradually, is quite severe but only with certain movements, and may be absent when lying down—until you try to turn. As with the other conditions described previously, facet joint irritation may cause pain that radiates down the ipsilateral leg. It rarely causes numbness or paresthesias in the leg.

Let's look at the simplified chart for a patient with facet joint irritation:

PHYSICAL EXAMINATION

Palpation	Findings resemble a sacroiliac ligament strain, with the big exception that the tenderness here is in the lumbar spine rather than over the sacroiliac joint. The pain may be localized directly over the irritated facet region, or it may be more diffuse. There may be a sciatic shift, and there may be spasm.
Range of Motion	Usually markedly restricted and quite painful.
Orthopaedic and Neurologic Tests	No signs of nerve root irritation because the nerve roots are not injured.

TESTS YOU MIGHT HAVE	WHAT THEY MIGHT SHOW
Lumbar Spine X-rays	Will usually appear normal. Hence, the injury can be attributed to an abnormal stress across the facet joint. So facet joint irritation can occur as a result of the abnormal rubbing of the facets during some activity.

Something else that occasionally shows on lumbar spine x-rays can sometimes pinpoint an irritated facet joint. Instead of finding all the facet joints aligned in a fairly straight line as we look up and down the lumbar spine on a front-view x-ray, we may see one facet joint on one side of one vertebra that is definitely out of alignment. (**Fig. 3–5**) It will angle inward from above to below. This actually happens in individuals with this abnormality while the spine is growing, and so is present from the end of adolescence onward. Usually, it doesn't cause any problem; but if you happen to bend or twist the wrong way, it will let you know you've done something bad.

MRI Scan and CAT Scan Studies

Will all be normal, as will EMGs and NCTs.

Figure 3-5

Rotated Facet Joints

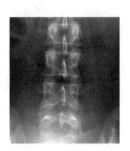
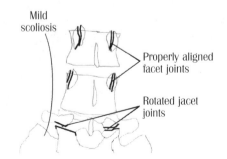

X-ray Vision

The bilateral rotated facets at the fifth lumbar vertebra on the front view x-ray on page 57 of the lower lumbar spine are virtually horizontal in orientation. They will function well when the patient flexes and extends (bends forward and backward) but may interfere with the ability to rotate (twist side to side). Notice that there is also a mild scoliosis, which actually extends all the way to the first lumbar vertebra.

As with ligament injuries, if the pseudo-symptoms in the leg are severe enough, the patient and doctor may be fooled into believing that there is nerve root irritation and/or a herniated disc.

Herniated Disc

Believe it or not, herniated discs (also called ruptured discs, slipped discs, or chipped discs) are responsible for only about 5 percent of episodes of lower back pain. We hear so much about them, and their symptoms can be so dramatic, that it seems as if they are a lot more prevalent than is really the case. Common causes of herniated lumbar discs are heavy lifting, incorrect lifting or carrying, bending, twisting, and sudden violent forward flexion (you fly forward after being tackled in a pickup football game or if you aren't wearing your seat belt in a motor vehicle accident). In fact, I treated one patient on two different occasions, each time after she'd herniated a different disc while playing tennis!

When a disc herniates, the nucleus pulposus (the cherry jelly) pushes back through the annulus fibrosus (the doughnut). Sometimes the annulus is tough enough that it keeps the nucleus from pushing all the way through it, but the annulus itself sticks out. (**Fig. 3–6**) Sometimes the nucleus extrudes all the way through the annulus. (**Fig. 3–7**)

Figure 3-6

Herniated Disc: Herniated Nucleus Pulposus with Intact Annulus Fibrosus

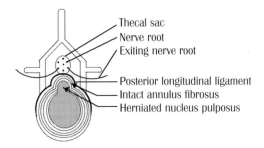

Thecal sac
Nerve root
Exiting nerve root

Posterior longitudinal ligament
Intact annulus fibrosus
Herniated nucleus pulposus

Figure 3-7

Herniated Disc: Herniated Nucleus Pulposus with Disrupted Annulus Fibrosus

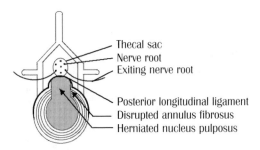

Thecal sac
Nerve root
Exiting nerve root

Posterior longitudinal ligament
Disrupted annulus fibrosus
Herniated nucleus pulposus

In both cases, the posterior longitudinal ligament will be forced upward off the back side of the disc and adjacent vertebral body. If the disc herniates with enough force, a part or all of the nucleus may literally explode through the annulus *and* tear through the posterior longitudinal ligament. That's called a **free fragment** and almost always causes dramatic symptoms because it frequently kinks the nerve root. (**Fig. 3–8**)

Figure 3-8

Herniated Disc with Free Fragment

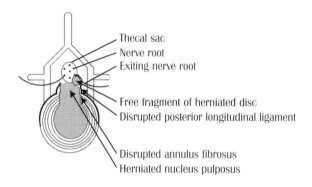

Thecal sac
Nerve root
Exiting nerve root

Free fragment of herniated disc
Disrupted posterior longitudinal ligament

Disrupted annulus fibrosus
Herniated nucleus pulposus

The pain with many lumbar disc herniations begins at the moment of injury. It is usually centered at the area corresponding to the location of the disc, although there are a few times when back pain is not the predominant symptom. Because the disc presses against a spinal nerve root, the nerve root is instantly irritated. This irritation is manifested as radiating pain along the course of the nerve root, which may start around the hip or buttock area and travel down the leg to the thigh, calf, ankle, or foot, depending on where in lumbar spine the nerve root originated. At the far end of the nerve root, there will often be pain, numbness, and/or paresthesias in the muscles and skin supplied by that nerve root. The general term used to describe irritation causing pain along the course of a nerve is **radiculopathy.** This is the condition that laypeople call a **pinched nerve**, and, in fact, the nerve is literally pinched, squeezed, or compressed. Coughing or sneezing may create sudden, excruciating pain in the low back, the leg, or both. In certain rare severe cases, the bowels or bladder may be affected.

It's important to understand that individual nerve roots don't actually travel alone from the spinal canal to the leg. Instead, groups of them join together and become a main nerve trunk. In chapter 1, you saw how the individual nerve roots exit on each side between the pedicles of adjacent vertebrae. In the lumbar spine, the nerve roots that exit at the second, third, and fourth lumbar vertebrae join together to form the **femoral nerve**, which then comes around to the front of the body and supplies all the muscles and skin on the front of the thigh. (**Fig. 3–9**)

Figure 3-9

Femoral Nerve and Its Roots

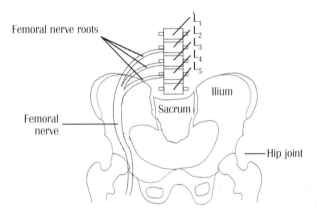

The femoral nerve is also responsible for the knee-jerk reflex (the patellar tendon reflex). The nerve roots that exit at the fourth and fifth lumbar vertebrae and from special areas of the first, second, and third sacral vertebrae (which are actually fused together) join together to form the **sciatic nerve**. (**Fig. 3–10**)

$$\mathcal{F}igure\ 3\text{-}10$$

Sciatic Nerve and Its Roots

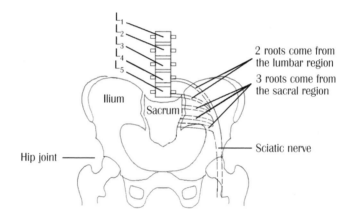

The sciatic nerve is as big around as your thumb. It supplies all the muscles on the back of the thigh (which are collectively called the hamstrings) and all the muscles of the entire calf, ankle, and foot with the ability to contract. It also supplies all the skin of those areas with sensation.

 Remember: Sensation is supplied by nerve roots in longitudinal bands called dermatomes.

The sciatic nerve is also responsible for the ankle-jerk reflex (the Achilles reflex). Because most herniated lumbar discs are at the lower end of the lumbar spine, they press against one of the lumbar nerve roots that will become part of the sciatic nerve. The term **sciatica** is used to describe the pain along the course of that nerve.

In addition to pain, numbness, and/or paresthesias, another symptom that may be associated with a herniated lumbar disc is a feeling of weakness in certain parts of the leg. If the disc presses on a nerve root going to the femoral nerve, a muscle or muscles on the front of the thigh may be weak, and the knee may feel as if it is going to buckle. If a nerve root to the sciatic nerve is affected, sometimes certain calf muscles will be weak and the foot will slap down on the ground when you walk. (This condition has the sensible medical name of "foot slap.")

PHYSICAL EXAMINATION

Inspection	May show no abnormality, or it may show a sciatic shift. (You can have a sciatic shift even if it's the femoral nerve that's irritated.)
Palpation	There may or may not be spasm; there may or may not be tenderness.
Range of Motion	Will usually be limited due to pain.
Orthopaedic and Neurologic Tests	Here's where the best information comes from.
	Sensation will frequently be diminished to light touch and pinprick in the dermatome associated with the irritated nerve root. A careful manual muscle exam will frequently demonstrate weakness of the muscle or muscles supplied by that nerve root. If the femoral nerve is the culprit, the knee-jerk reflex (patellar tendon) will often be diminished or absent. If the sciatic nerve

is involved—specifically if the nerve root exiting between the fifth lumbar and first sacral vertebrae is irritated—the Achilles (ankle-jerk or gastro-soleus) reflex will be diminished or absent.

<u>TESTS YOU MIGHT HAVE</u>	<u>WHAT THEY MIGHT SHOW</u>
Lumbar Spine X-rays	Plane lumbar spine x-rays, of course, will only show the bones, so they're not going to be of any real diagnostic value.
MRI Scan and CAT Scan Studies	An MRI scan of the lumbar spine will show the disc literally pressing on the nerve root. (**Fig. 3–11**) A CAT scan of the lumbar spine should show the same things as the MRI scan, though with a different kind of detail. (**Fig. 3–12**)
Lumbar Myelogram	Will also show a herniated disc—but by inference. Remember: A myelogram involves injecting dye inside the covering that surrounds the spinal nerve roots. If a disc is herniated and pressing on a nerve root, it will indent it; that indentation of the dye is what we see. (**Fig. 3–13**)
Lumbar Discogram	May also show a herniated disc, especially if it is one that resulted in a free fragment. If the discogram needle is properly centered in the nucleus and the nucleus has herniated, then the dye that's injected will flow out into the annulus and, if the posterior

longitudinal ligament is torn, out into the spinal canal. (**Fig. 3–14**)

EMGs and NCTs   Can help to make the diagnosis as well. Unfortunately, it takes about three weeks after an insult to a nerve root for signs of nerve root irritation to show up on EMGs. The results can be quite impressive: We can see a variety of changes that are limited just to the muscles supplied by the injured nerve root. The NCTs will often show that the specific nerve root itself is not functioning normally.

Figure 3-11

MRI Scan Showing Herniated Disc

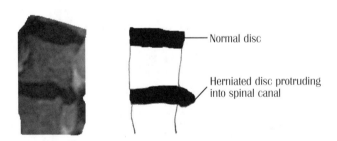

Normal disc

Herniated disc protruding into spinal canal

X-ray Vision

This disc is markedly herniated and severely indents the thecal sac. Compare the posterior herniation to the flat posterior edge of the disc one level above.

Figure 3-12

CAT Scan Showing Herniated Disc

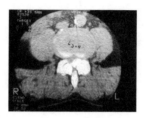

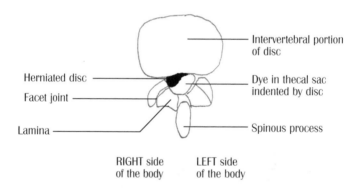

Intervertebral portion of disc

Herniated disc

Facet joint

Lamina

Dye in thecal sac indented by disc

Spinous process

RIGHT side
of the body

LEFT side
of the body

X-ray Vision

To keep you on your toes, note that the left side of the picture is actually the right side of the body (note the "R" at the bottom left of the CAT scan), and that the right side of the picture is actually the left side of the body (note the "L" at the bottom right of the CAT scan).

This is a special CAT scan that was done just after the patient had had a myelogram, so the dye is still inside the thecal sac. That allows us to see exactly how the disc is herniated on the right side and how it has indented and pushed the thecal sac toward the left.

Figure 3-13

Myelogram Showing Herniated Disc

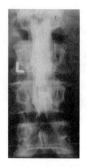

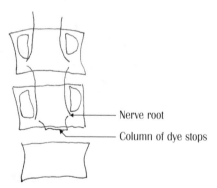

Nerve root

Column of dye stops

X-ray Vision

This front view shows that the column of dye suddenly stops. That's because this herniated disc is so huge that it not only indents a nerve root, it completely indents the thecal sac and constricts it so much that there is no room for dye to flow between the thecal sac and the nerve roots inside it.

Figure 3-14

Discograms Showing Herniated Disc

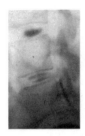
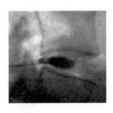

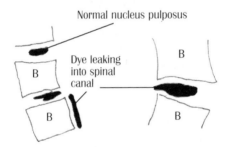

B=Vertebral body

X-ray Vision

These discograms show exactly what was depicted in Figure 3-8: The nucleus pulposus has burst through both the annulus fibrosus and the posterior longitudinal ligament. The dye leaking into the spinal canal means that there is a free fragment of disc lying in the canal. In both of these studies, the height of the disc space is normal and the thickness of the vertebral end plates (the flat surfaces of the ends of the vertebral bodies that abut against the disc) is normal, meaning that the disc had not previously degenerated. We'll learn more about that in chapter 4.

Compression Fracture

Falling from a height, jumping from a height, attempting to push up to try to open a really stuck window, or getting violently bent forward (as when being tackled in a football game or being in a motor vehicle accident when wearing a seat belt but not a shoulder harness) can all cause the same kind of injury: a compression fracture of a lumbar vertebral body. This results in a simple wedge-shaped deformity if it is a simple compression fracture. The anterior (front) part of the vertebral body compresses, while the posterior (back) edge of the body usually maintains its length. (**Fig. 3–15**)

Figure 3-15

X-ray Showing Compression Fracture

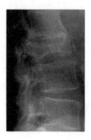

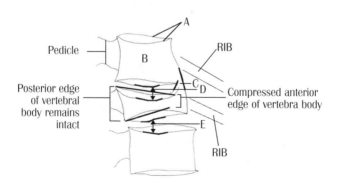

X-ray Vision

We can clearly see how the compression of the anterior (front) portion of the vertebral body has resulted in a wedge-shaped deformity in the x-ray on page 69. But remember that this lateral (side-view) x-ray is a 2-dimensional flat representation of the actual 3-dimensional vertebral body, which is a cylinder. Thus we see the front and back edges of the top of the cylinder (the vertebral end plate) as separate lines **(A)** because the x-ray beam wasn't aimed directly across the top of the vertebral body. The same thing occurs at each vertebral end plate.

A bony bridge **(C)** has formed between the fractured vertebra and the one above **(B)** when the blood that had leaked out anteriorly at the time of the fracture later turned to bone. Note that the discs above **(D)** and below **(E)** the fractured vertebra remained intact and did not collapse: the heights of the disc spaces are normal.

The pain is immediate, often intense, localized, unremitting, present even at rest, increased with attempting to roll over, and either sharp or dull. There usually is no radiating pain, numbness, or paresthesias.

Take a look at our chart:

Physical Examination

Palpation	Tenderness and spasm.
Percussion	Marked tenderness.
Range of Motion	Restricted. Actually, if a compression fracture is suspected, it's best to have the patient lie down and avoid any kind of range of motion.

Orthopaedic and Neurologic Tests

With a simple compression fracture, there usually are no changes. If the compression fracture has been more extensive, with pieces of bone breaking off and going through the posterior longitudinal ligament into the spinal canal, the symptoms and physical examination will be as dramatic as with an acutely herniated disc.

<u>**TESTS YOU MIGHT HAVE**</u>

<u>**WHAT THEY MIGHT SHOW**</u>

Lumbar Spine X-rays

Will show a compression fracture of the vertebral body.

MRI Scan and CAT Scan Studies

An MRI scan will show the compression fracture and bleeding in the marrow of the vertebral body. (**Fig. 3–16**) It may actually show a tear of the posterior longitudinal ligament. It will show blood and possibly debris in the spinal canal, and it will show any kinking or impingement on the thecal sac (the covering of the spinal cord and spinal nerve roots). A CAT scan will also show the compression fracture and thecal sac indentation.

Three-phase Bone Scan

Will show dye throughout the body of the compressed vertebra. (**Fig. 3–17**)

EMGs and NCTs

Negative if the compression fracture is a simple one with no disruption of the posterior part of the vertebral body.

Figure 3-16

MRI Scan Showing Compression Fracture

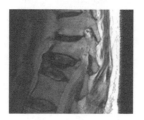

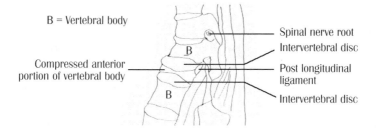

B = Vertebral body

Compressed anterior
portion of vertebral body

B

B

Spinal nerve root

Intervertebral disc

Post longitudinal
ligament

Intervertebral disc

X-ray Vision

The posterior longitudinal ligament remained intact, so no bony fragments entered the spinal canal. The vertebral body compressed, but
the intervertebral discs above and below the compressed vertebra remained intact, and their heights are normal. We can also see a spinal
nerve root in the intervertebral foramen.

Figure 3-17

Bone Scans Showing Compression Fractures

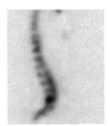

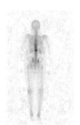

Compression fracture
of L_5 lateral view

Compression fracture
of T_{12} front view

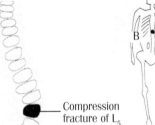

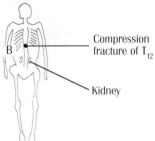

Compression
fracture of T_{12}

Kidney

Compression
fracture of L_5

X-ray Vision

At three hours, the radioactive dye has been evenly distributed through-out the entire body, giving us the classic picture of a skeleton on the front view. The dye gets concentrated at the site of the compression fracture, which is why it looks so black. The dye gets removed from the body by the kidneys, which also concentrate it. That's why they are as dark as the compression fracture.

Painful Coccyx

The coccyx consists of four very small bones at the very bottom of the spine. It is located low between the buttocks (the intergluteal cleft). Laypeople call it the tailbone, and the coccygeal bones *are* the bones of the tail in animals. The coccyx serves no real function in humans; in fact, people function equally well even if the coccyx has been removed. An injured coccyx can be the source of intense pain and can cause marked discomfort far out of proportion to its diminutive size.

The coccyx can be injured when you slip and fall and land directly on the buttocks. This can result either in a contusion (a bruise) or a fracture. The coccyx can also be fractured during childbirth. The pain comes on rapidly, is located exactly at the base of the spine, and does not radiate anywhere.

Here is what our chart shows:

PHYSICAL EXAMINATION

Palpation	Exquisite tenderness directly over the coccyx. There will not be any spasm or flattening of lordosis during flexion.
Range of Motion	May be restricted by pain.
Orthopaedic and Neurologic Tests	Normal.

TESTS YOU MIGHT HAVE · WHAT THEY MIGHT SHOW

Lumbar Spine X-rays	Will be normal if the coccyx is only contused, or will show a fracture of the coccyx.

Chapter Four

CHRONIC CONDITIONS
WHAT THEY ARE AND HOW WE FIND THEM

In this chapter, you'll learn about painful episodes caused by some change that has slowly taken place in the structures of the low back. These changes may occur in bones, joints, ligaments, and/or discs. Because they come on very gradually—taking anywhere from one year to a lifetime—they don't cause pain as they are developing. Instead, pain arises when something suddenly happens to cause irritation. There are a number of such conditions.

Degenerative Disc Disease

I described in chapter 1 how discs lose some of their water content as they age and that this process may begin as early as age fifteen. Some young people's discs look like they're seventy years old, some people over the age of sixty have discs that look like a twenty-year-old's, and some people's discs age in concert with their chronologic age.

 Remember: The water content of a disc is contained in the nucleus (the cherry jelly) and is responsible for its resilience.

When a disc starts to lose some of its water, it's less resilient. It doesn't act as well as it used to in serving as a shock absorber. The nucleus shrivels as water is lost, reducing the height of the disc—and thus the width of the space between one vertebra and the next (which is called the interspace). (**Fig. 4–1**)

Figure 4 - 1

X-rays Showing Degenerative Disc Disease

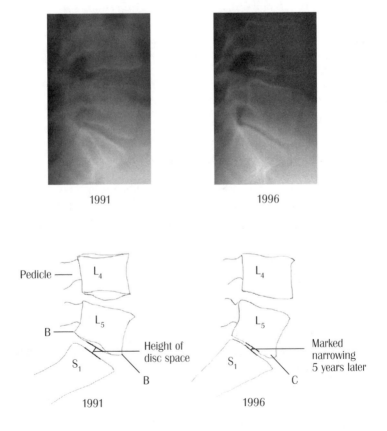

X-ray Vision

Note that in the x-rays on page 76, in 1991 this disc has actually already started to degenerate. We see that the disc space is narrower than the two disc spaces above. There is no change in the thickness of the pedicle.

This is the appearance **(B)** of the corners of a vertebra just as spurs start to form, and as they continue to develop **(C)**.

The flat end surfaces of the bodies of the vertebrae on each side of a degenerated disc—the **vertebral end plates**—will gradually react to the loss of resilience the disc formerly provided. The reaction consists of thickening or enlarging, a condition known as **hypertrophy**. If you hold a small, round piece of soft clay between your two palms and slowly compress it, it will expand circumferentially as it gets compressed. The same thing happens to an aging disc. As it loses its water and narrows, it simultaneously expands circumferentially, or **bulges**. As it does so, the posterior and anterior longitudinal ligaments are pushed outward, and the circumferential edge of the vertebral end plates gets pulled out as well. **(Fig. 4–2)**

Figure 4-2

"Blueprint" Views of Disc Narrowing and Spurs

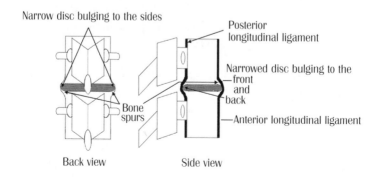

Narrow disc bulging to the sides

Posterior longitudinal ligament

Narrowed disc bulging to the —front and —back

Bone spurs

Anterior longitudinal ligament

Back view   Side view

We can see that outward projection of the bony vertebral end plate; you might have heard it called a **spur**.

Degenerative disc disease may be irritated by any type of activity, or it may never be irritated by activity! If it *is* irritated by an activity such as bending, lifting, twisting, or the like, it will cause symptoms of lower back pain that may be mild, moderate, or severe; may be constant or intermittent; may be increased with certain activities; and frequently subside with rest. Sometimes this may be accompanied by pain in one or both legs, either just in the hip area or continuing down the leg. Rarely will patients experience numbness or paresthesias or an increase in symptoms with coughing and sneezing.

Here's what a simplified chart might look like for a patient with degenerative disc disease:

PHYSICAL EXAMINATION

Inspection	Nothing abnormal.
Palpation	Some tenderness observed. (Many doctors think they feel spasm, but as I said earlier, that's something that is overdiagnosed in this condition.)
Range of Motion	Limited in one or several directions; often accompanied by pain, and sometimes by segmental spasm.
Orthopaedic and Neurologic Tests	Almost always normal.

TESTS YOU MIGHT HAVE

WHAT THEY MIGHT SHOW

Lumbar Spine X-rays

The disc is invisible on plane x-rays, but if the x-rays show narrowing of the space where the disc should be, we know the disc has degenerated. We will often also see bone spurs at the edge of the vertebral end plates and, if the process has been going on for a long time, thickening of the vertebral end plates.

MRI Scan

The MRI can show loss of water in the disc, narrowing of the disc (and thus of the interspace), thickening of the vertebral end plates, hypertrophic bony spurring, and bulging of the disc either asymmetrically or partially or fully circumferentially. **(Fig. 4–3)**

Figure 4-3

MRI Scan Showing Bulging Disc

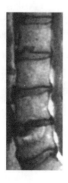
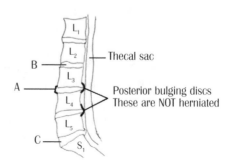

X-ray Vision

The disc between the third and fourth lumbar vertebrae actually bulges circumferentially. We see it protruding anteriorly toward the abdominal cavity **(A)** as well as posteriorly. We can also see the **thecal sac,** which is the covering of the central group of spinal nerve roots in the spinal canal. Note that the two bulging discs are narrower in height than the discs at **(B)** and **(C),** which are not degenerated.

Junior Doctor's Merit Badge Checkpoint

You might think that the bulging of the disc described above is significant, but you'd be wrong. Let me explain why.

If you saw a photograph of a man with graying hair and some wrinkles around the eyes, I don't think you'd say, "Oh, he must be very sick!" Instead, I think you'd say, "He looks as if he's getting a little older." I also believe that you wouldn't think that those changes of gray hair and some wrinkles around the eyes had just occurred a day or two before the picture was taken.

Well, a lumbar spine MRI scan—or a CAT scan—is actually just a picture of the lumbar spine, and it shows the same signs of aging inside the body that a photograph shows of the outside. A bulging disc and its accompanying bone spurs are nothing more than signs of aging (*except* in some cases of **spinal stenosis**, which you'll learn about later). If the disc only bulges, and does not impinge upon, indent, or displace a spinal nerve root, the disc cannot cause leg symptoms of any kind. Degenerative bulging of a disc won't cause any nerve root irritation if the disc hasn't come in contact with a nerve root, so EMGs and NCTs will be normal. **(Fig. 4–4)**

Figure 4-4

MRI Cross Section Showing Bulging Disc

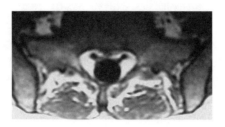

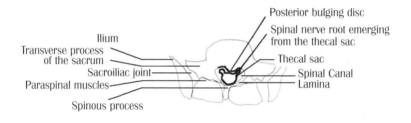

Posterior bulging disc

Spinal nerve root emerging from the thecal sac

Ilium

Transverse process of the sacrum

Sacroiliac joint

Paraspinal muscles

Spinous process

Thecal sac

Spinal Canal

Lamina

X-ray Vision

Neither the thecal sac nor the exiting spinal nerve root are touched, impinged upon, or indented by the bulging disc. It's literally as if the disc were a mile away: It can't cause symptoms. This cross section is oriented 180° from the "Blueprint" Top Views in chapter 1, so the abdominal cavity is toward the top and the skin of the back is toward the bottom.

This disc is actually between the fifth lumbar and first sacral vertebrae. How do we know? We can see the big hip bone, the ilium, the transverse process of the sacrum, and the sacroiliac joint. We can also see the paraspinal muscles, the spinous process, the spinal canal, and the lamina.

Sometimes, when a disc degenerates, it does so asymmetrically in one of several ways. As we just saw above, it may bulge just to one side rather than circumferentially across the back of the vertebral body. A more dramatic form of asymmetric disc degeneration occurs when one whole side of the disc shrivels or collapses. This results in greater narrowing of one side of the intervertebral disc space compared to the other side. As a result, the vertebra above is tilted toward the narrowed side. This can actually cause a tilting of the lumbar spine above that level, which is, in turn, often accompanied by asymmetric degeneration *on the opposite side* of a disc higher up. The end result is then a mild **degenerative scoliosis**. (**Fig. 4–5**) Sometimes the asymmetric narrowing will lead to spur formation and nerve root impingement, which you'll learn about in the next section.

When the degeneration of a disc continues for a long period of time, usually over several years and usually—but not always—after middle age, the water that was contained in the nucleus pulposus, but evaporated, is replaced by nitrogen gas. The nitrogen gas is a lousy shock absorber. We can see evidence of replacement of water by nitrogen gas in a nucleus pulposus on a routine x-ray. The intervertebral disc space will look very black (because the x-ray beam passes through nitrogen more easily than it does through water). We call this x-ray appearance of the black interspace a **vacuum disc phenomenon**. (**Fig. 4–6**)

Degenerative Arthritis

Just as the discs can wear as we age, so can the vertebrae and facet joints.

Greek Lesson

Technically speaking, the term arthritis refers only to joints—it's Greek and means "inflammation of a joint." We bend the grammar rule slightly in the spine and use the term arthritis to refer not only to changes in the facet joints but also to thickening or spur formation of the pedicles.

Figure 4-5

X-ray Showing Asymmetric Disc Degeneration

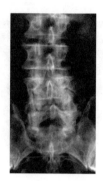

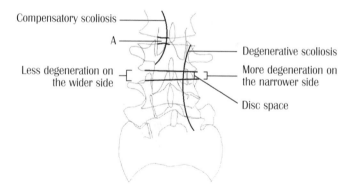

Compensatory scoliosis

A

Less degeneration on
the wider side

Degenerative scoliosis

More degeneration on
the narrower side

Disc space

X-ray Vision

The marked degeneration of the disc on the right has resulted in a degenerative scoliosis centered at that area. As a result, there is narrowing on the opposite side **(A)** of the disc that's one level above the area of marked asymmetric disc degeneration. This has, in turn, resulted in a *compensatory scoliosis* centered at **(A)** that curves to the opposite side. The net effect is that the overall alignment of the spine stays straight.

Figure 4-6

X-ray Showing Vacuum Disc

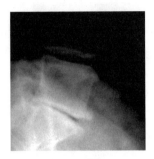

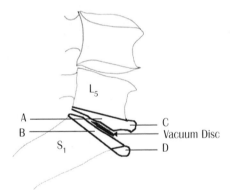

X-ray Vision

A vacuum disc represents the last stage of disc degeneration. The complete loss of water from the nucleus pulposus causes a tremendous reaction in the bones on each side of that disc. We can see that reaction as marked thickening of the vertebral end plates of the vertebrae above **(A)** and below **(B)** the degenerated disc and by the formation of large bone spurs above **(C)** and below **(D)** anteriorly (in front).

We know that joints—the surfaces of side-by-side (or **apposing**) bones that face each other—may become arthritic with age. This means that their ultrasmooth surfaces, which consist of a covering layer called **cartilage** that's far smoother than Teflon, become roughened. Some of the cartilage may actually wear away. Cartilage is not bone; the main difference is that cartilage has no blood vessels or calcium in it, so it's invisible on an x-ray.

 Remember: Only structures with calcium in them show up on plane x-rays.

If cartilage has worn away, then the space will be narrower between the two apposing bones at a joint. We *can* see this narrowing of the joint space on an x-ray; when we do, we can infer that arthritis is present. As the facet joint cartilage wears away, the forces transmitted across the facet joint become too great for it. The facet joint reacts in a misguided fashion. It tries to increase its surface area, or **hypertrophy**, to reduce the force per unit of surface area. But the new bone that forms to create this increased surface area is irregularly thickened. It's a bone spur, and can be called a **hypertrophic spur**. This process occurs very slowly—over a period of several years. (**Fig. 4–7**)

Bending and lifting can place tremendous stresses on the spine. For example, if you hold your arm outstretched in front of you, the distance from your hand to a line down the center of your lumbar vertebral bodies is fifteen times the distance from the center of the lumbar vertebral bodies to the tip of the lumbar spinous processes. This means that, for every pound you lift with your outstretched hand, there's a force of *15 pounds per square inch* over the lower lumbar discs. That force gets transmitted across the pedicles as the paraspinal muscles contract to keep you upright while you're lifting. Over a period of many years, the pedicles may thicken as a result.

Figure 4-7

X-ray Showing Facet Arthritis

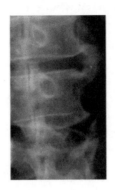

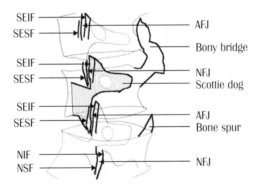

SEIF = Sclerotic edge of inferior facet
SESF = Sclerotic edge of superior facet
NIF = Normal edge of inferior facet
NSF = Normal edge of superior facet
AFJ = Abnormal facet joint
NFJ = Normal facet joint

X-ray Vision

On the x-ray on page 86, as you compare the width of the normal facet joint with the narrow spaces of the arthritic facet joints above, you also see how thick (or **sclerotic**) are the apposing edges of the arthritic facets. Note that the inferior facet comes from the lamina while the superior facet comes from the pedicle.

Notice also the enormous bony bridge that has formed as a result of spur formation that has enlarged over a period of many years. A second spur has also begun to form lower down.

In the Preface, I told you about the lady who had Scottie dog trouble. We'll learn about the Scottie dog later in this chapter. This x-ray is a *oblique view:* a view in which the patient is turned partly to the side, like a door that's ajar rather than fully open or closed.

Degenerative arthritis of the spine is thus due to the wear and tear of the passage of time. It results in a variety of symptoms. These include stiffness—the feeling that the back just doesn't want to bend when you first get up from bed or after sitting for a while—aching, pain and stiffness when bending over, pain that seems to be worse in damp or cold weather, and so on. Degenerative arthritis of the spine does not affect the spinal nerve roots, and so there will be no neurologic symptoms of numbness, paresthesias, or weakness. If degenerative arthritis of the spine progresses, however, it can cause serious neurologic problems, which you'll learn about in the next section on spinal stenosis.

Here's a simplified chart for a patient with degenerative arthritis:

PHYSICAL EXAMINATION

Inspection	Possibly some loss of lordosis.
Palpation	No particularly tender area.
Range of Motion	Stiffness or reduced motion, especially in flexion and extension, as well as lack of reversal of lordosis on forward flexion; range of motion may also be accompanied by pain.
Orthopaedic and Neurologic Tests	Normal.

 Remember: Flexion is bending forward; extension is bending backward.

TESTS YOU MIGHT HAVE	WHAT THEY MIGHT SHOW
Lumbar Spine X-rays	Spurring of the facets and/or pedicles.
MRI Scan and CAT Scan Studies	These studies will also show the bony spurring, while confirming that the spurs do not touch (we use the word *impinge*) the nerve roots or thecal sac.
EMGs and NCTs	Will be normal because the nerve roots are not irritated.

Spinal Stenosis

Sometimes posterior bulging of the disc and the accompanying thickening of the posterior longitudinal ligament and the posterior aspect of the vertebral body can also be accompanied by degenerative changes involving the facets and pedicles (the walls of the spinal house) and even by thickening of the underside of the ligamentum flavum (the interlaminar yellow ligament). When several or all of these things become thickened or hypertrophied, they narrow the diameter of the spinal canal. That's a condition called **spinal stenosis**. (**Fig. 4–8**) By itself, it would mean nothing and would not cause any symptoms.

Figure 4-8

MRI Cross Sections Showing Normal Spine and Spinal Stenosis

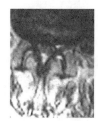
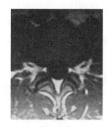

Normal   Spinal stenosis

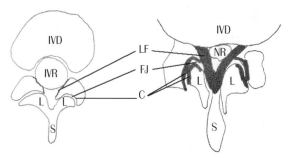

IVD = Intervertebral disc
NR = Nerve roots
L = Lamina
S = Spinous process
FJ = Facet joint
LF = Ligamentum flavum
C = Cartilage

X-ray Vision

The spinal nerve roots in the normal MRI scan on page 89 are contained in the thecal sac, which looks like a circle. But in the vertebra with spinal stenosis, the ligamentum flavum is markedly thickened, the facet joints are much more vertically oriented, the cartilage lining the facet joints is thickened (making facet joint arthritis) and the thecal sac is compressed and distorted. As a result, it looks like a lima bean.

But the spinal canal is the home of the central group of spinal nerve roots contained within their covering, the **thecal sac** (another name for this covering is the **dura**), and of the individual nerve roots that exit between each pair of vertebrae. The exiting nerve roots go between adjacent pedicles, and the space through which they go is called the **intervertebral foramen** or **neural foramen**. (You saw an MRI scan showing the intervertebral foramina and exiting nerve roots in chapter 1, figure 1–23.)

Latin Lesson

Foramen is the Latin word for opening or hole. Just to keep you on your toes, one is a foramen; two are foramina. Yes, the *e* gets changed to an *i*. Those Romans were such jokesters!

If spinal stenosis progresses to the point that any or all of these thickened structures touch the thecal sac and/or the exiting nerve root or roots, that *can* be a serious problem akin to a herniated disc. Symptoms may include constant and unremitting back pain (a dull, nagging ache that just doesn't go away), radiating leg pain that may be constant or intermittent and that sometimes feels like a gnawing pain (like when you dig a knuckle into the skin and turn it back and forth), paresthesias, numbness, and weakness.

You might also have **spinal** or **neurogenic claudication**, which means that the leg or buttock pain comes on when you extend your back.

Take a look at a simplified chart for a patient with spinal stenosis:

PHYSICAL EXAMINATION

Inspection	Possibly loss of lordosis.
Palpation	No immediate tenderness, but there may be tenderness on percussion over the spinous processes of the affected vertebrae.
Range of Motion	Often restricted, and extension often reproduces the symptoms of pain and even paresthesias and numbness.
Orthopaedic and Neurologic Tests	May show decreased sensation and sometimes muscle weakness. Reflexes may be diminished.

 Remember: Percussion is tapping over a specific area.

TESTS YOU MIGHT HAVE	**WHAT THEY MIGHT SHOW**
Lumbar Spine X-rays	Bony spurring of vertebral end plates, pedicles, foramina, and laminae.
MRI Scan and CAT Scan Studies	Will also show those same bony changes as well as thickening of the ligamentum flavum (which is, of course, invisible on a plane x-ray) in cross-sectional pictures. In addition, these studies also show the thecal sac and exiting nerve roots and will show actual indentation by hypertrophic structures. (**Fig. 4–9**)

TESTS YOU MIGHT HAVE	**WHAT THEY MIGHT SHOW**
Myelogram **EMGs and NCTs**	Indentation or kinking of the thecal sac. May show signs of irritated muscles and nerves similar to findings with a herniated disc. This may help distinguish spinal claudication from another condition called **vascular claudication**, which is pain and cramping in the legs—especially the calves—with activity and walking. Vascular claudication comes from poor circulation and has nothing to do with the spine or the nerve roots. Its treatment is quite different from the treatment of spinal claudication.

Figure 4-9

MRI Scan Showing Spinal Stenosis

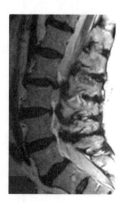

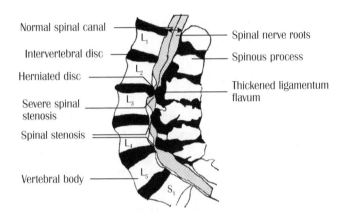

Normal spinal canal — L₁
Intervertebral disc —
Herniated disc — L₂
Severe spinal stenosis — L₃
Spinal stenosis — L₄
Vertebral body — L₅ S₁

Spinal nerve roots
Spinous process
Thickened ligamentum flavum

X-ray Vision

Note how the intervertebral disc between the second and third lumbar vertebrae protrudes both anteriorly (toward the front) and posteriorly into the spinal canal on the MRI scan on page 92. In fact, this disc has herniated into the spinal canal and markedly indents the spinal nerve roots. The ligamentum flavum at that same level has also markedly thickened and protrudes dramatically into the spinal canal directly opposite the herniated disc. That's what has so severely constricted the spinal nerve roots, causing the tremendous spinal stenosis there. At the next two levels below, between the third and fourth lumbar vertebrae and between the fourth and fifth lumbar vertebrae, the ligamentum flavum has again markedly thickened, but the posterior portions of the intervertebral discs have not bulged into the spinal canal, so the spinal stenosis there is not quite as severe, although it is still extensive.

Stress Fracture

Gymnasts, swim team divers, weight lifters, and other athletes may be susceptible to spinal stress fractures. You know how, if you fall and break a bone, the bone snaps immediately and breaks instantly? Well that's just what a stress fracture is *not*! A stress fracture occurs when a bone very gradually weakens from *frequently* repeated stresses to it. Individual bone cells get disrupted and die. More and more do so over a period of time, to the point that, eventually, enough bone cells die to create a linear disruption in the bone. The bone may ultimately crack all the way across to become a genuine fracture.

The symptoms of a stress fracture come on slowly. Initially, you might feel only mild, intermittent episodes of pain. These gradually become more frequent, and in time they become a continuous pain that may be deep and gnawing. This pain usually increases with activity and eases with rest.

Let's look at a simplified chart for a patient with a stress fracture:

PHYSICAL EXAMINATION

Palpation	Tenderness and spasm.
Percussion	Tenderness.
Range of Motion	Tenderness and possibly segmental spasm.
Orthopaedic and Neurologic Tests	No abnormalities.

TESTS YOU MIGHT HAVE · WHAT THEY MIGHT SHOW

Lumbar Spine X-rays	May be negative (normal) in the early stages of a stress fracture. If the fracture has been present long enough, then x-rays may show

the line of the fracture and, frequently, some thickening of the bone immediately adjacent to the line. This thickening, which is called **sclerosis**, is caused by a reaction of the bone immediately adjacent to the stress fracture. Extra bone is literally made by the body as a reaction to the slowly propagating fracture line, and so we can call it **reactive sclerosis**.

MRI Scan and CAT Scan Studies

An MRI can show a stress fracture in its relatively early stages because the MRI scan is such a sensitive indicator of the water content of bone, and a fracture has no water in it, while the early reactive sclerosis will be manifested by an increased blood supply bringing more calcium to the area. A CAT scan is usually not nearly as good for picking up an early stress fracture, though it will certainly show one that's been present for a while.

Three-phase Bone Scan

This is the nicest and simplest test for detecting a stress fracture—even an early one. The blood pool and three-hour films are excellent for showing the characteristic blood flow changes that are the signature of a stress fracture. (**Fig. 4–10**)

Developmental Bone Problems

Remember back in the introduction, I talked about a lady who was told she had problems with her Scottie Dogs, but she didn't have any dogs at home? She was actually talking about a developmental bone problem. These are abnormalities of the spinal bones that either are present at

birth or develop during the growth years or later in adulthood. A bony
condition that's present at birth is called a **congenital anomaly**. Congenital bone conditions are usually *not* hereditary—that is, they're not
passed from one generation to the next by the genes. Instead, they're
merely due to some tiny variation from the normal way a fetus should
develop. Other abnormalities may arise in children during their growth
years. And, boy, do they get fancy names!

Figure 4-10

Bone Scan Showing Stress Fracture

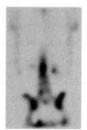

Front view

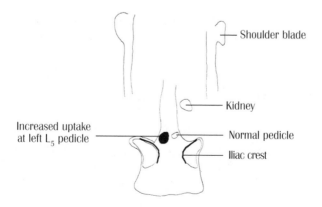

Shoulder blade

Kidney

Increased uptake
at left L$_5$ pedicle

Normal pedicle

Iliac crest

X-ray Vision

The bone scan on page 96 shows a stress fracture of the left pedicle of the fifth lumbar vertebra. The bone scan was positive weeks before the stress fracture could be seen on an x-ray.

Since the dye concentrates in bone containing a concentration of blood, we see the dye in the iliac crest and in the scapula, or shoulder blade, both of which have marrow that makes blood cells. The kidney is also visible because it concentrates the dye and excretes it.

SPONDYLOLYSIS

Spondylolysis is a Greek word meaning "the absence of spinal bone." Some people have spondylolysis as a congenital anomaly; others develop it in childhood or adolescence. It's an absence of bone in a special part of the pedicle (the pillar, or wall of our spinal "house"); that special area is called the **pars interarticularis**.

Latin Lesson

Pars interarticularis is Latin for the part between the anterior and posterior facet joints. Just to show you how those ancient Romans could toy with your mind, the plural is partes interarticulares.

Spondylolysis may not cause any symptoms for many years, and in fact may never cause symptoms. Sometimes, however, it may cause symptoms in adolescence or anytime in adulthood. Once it's there, it's there: Additional bone doesn't melt away as years pass. Usually it's present on both pedicles of one vertebra, and then it is called **bilateral spondylolysis**. If it's just present on one side, it may actually have begun as an undetected stress fracture. The one-sided condition, **unilateral spondylolysis,** is much less common than the bilateral form. Symptoms may include vague, intermittent lower back pain, while sometimes the pain may become constant and relieved by rest. Activities usually don't increase symptoms—except if activities include strenuous athletics or strenuous manual labor. There are usually no leg symptoms.

Take a look at the simplified chart for spondylolysis:

Physical Examination

Palpation	Localized tenderness over the affected vertebra; there may or may not be spasm.
Range of Motion	Usually normal; rarely will there be segmental spasm.
Orthopaedic and Neurologic Tests	Normal nerve function.

Tests You Might Have	What They Might Show
Lumbar Spine X-rays	Lumbar spine x-rays will instantly show the problem. When these x-rays are taken, they consist of a front (or back, if you prefer) view, a side view (called a lateral view), and two more views of the patient turned partway to each side (called oblique views). It's on the oblique view that part of the vertebra looks like a Scottie dog: The anterior facet is its ear, the transverse process is its nose, the pars interarticularis is its neck, the posterior facet is its foreleg, and the lamina

is its body. Spondylolysis on the oblique x-ray looks as if the Scottie dog has a broken or absent neck! **(Fig. 4–11)**

MRI Scan and Cat Scan Studies

These tests will show the problem, **(Fig. 4–12)** but they're not needed unless there's a reasonable concern that there's some nerve root or other problem present.

EMGs and NCTs

The absence of any nerve problems means these studies will be normal.

Figure 4-11

X-ray Showing Spondylolysis (Scottie Dog with "Broken Neck")

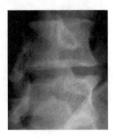

Oblique view

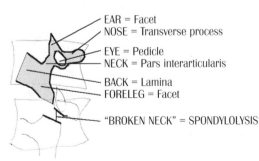

EAR = Facet
NOSE = Transverse process
EYE = Pedicle
NECK = Pars interarticularis
BACK = Lamina
FORELEG = Facet
"BROKEN NECK" = SPONDYLOLYSIS

X-ray Vision

The x-ray on page 99 is an oblique (partly turned) view. Sometimes, in young patients between the ages of six and sixteen, we can see a Scottie dog's "neck" start to narrow. If we take x-rays over a period of years, we may see it completely disappear. Once it's gone, it never reappears.

Figure 4-12

CAT Scan Showing Bilateral Spondylolysis

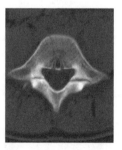

Cross section view

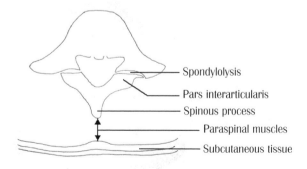

Spondylolysis

Pars interarticularis

Spinous process

Paraspinal muscles

Subcutaneous tissue

X-ray Vision

The CAT scan on page 100 clearly shows how there is a complete absence of bone and cartilage at the area of spondylolysis.

Notice the considerable thickness of the paraspinal muscles between the thin subcutaneous tissue and the spinous process. This patient was very muscular.

SPONDYLOLISTHESIS

This mouthful of a term is also Greek and means "slipping or dislocation of spinal bone." In order to have spondylolisthesis, you first need to have complete bilateral spondylolysis of both partes interarticulares of a vertebra. When that happens, the parts of the vertebra anterior to (in front of) the absent Scottie dog's neck—the vertebral body, intervertebral disc, anterior and posterior longitudinal ligaments, lowest parts of the pedicles—are no longer connected to the posterior (back) half of the vertebra—the transverse processes, upper half of the pedicles, laminae, spinous process, and the intertransverse and interspinous ligaments and ligamentum flavum.

As the years go by, from all the activities of life, the anterior half of the vertebra very slowly pulls away from the posterior half and slips forward. The anterior and posterior longitudinal ligaments and intervertebral disc keep the slipping anterior half firmly connected to the body of the next higher vertebra. Because of some special laws of physics, the disc between the slipping vertebra and the intact vertebra just below it tends to flatten and roll posteriorly into the spinal canal. That, along with the fact that the body of the vertebra may slip forward anywhere from a few millimeters to more than a full centimeter, means that the spinal nerve roots and their covering, the thecal sac, may be kinked. The associated exiting nerve roots may also be stretched. (**Fig. 4–13**)

Figure 4-13

Spondylolisthesis

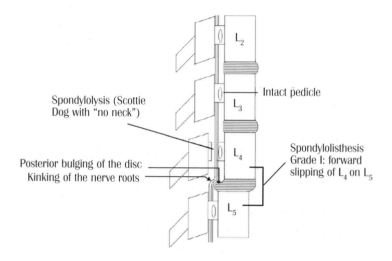

Spondylolysis (Scottie Dog with "no neck")

Posterior bulging of the disc
Kinking of the nerve roots

L₂

Intact pedicle

L₃

L₄

Spondylolisthesis
Grade I: forward
slipping of L₄ on L₅

L₅

Spondylolisthesis may begin in adolescence, but it usually starts in early adulthood. In the most extreme cases—which, fortunately, are very rare—the vertebral body slips so far forward that it literally falls off in front of the vertebral body below. That's a back problem way beyond the scope of this book. Spondylolisthesis is graded based on the percentage of the slipping of the vertebral body in relation to the one below. Up to a 25 percent slip is Grade I, a 25 to 50 percent slip is Grade II, and so forth. Spondylolisthesis is most commonly seen between the fourth and fifth lumbar vertebrae and between the fifth lumbar and first sacral vertebrae.

Spondylolisthesis is often painless. Frequently, it's only discovered when lumbar spine x-rays are taken for some other reason. Part of the reason is that since it's such a slowly occurring condition, the body has plenty of time to adapt to it and accommodate it. Sometimes, however, it may become painful, with constant low back ache and even some pain radiating down the legs. Rarely are there any symptoms of nerve root irritation. Activity may sometimes accentuate symptoms, and rest will relieve them.

Here's the simplified chart for this condition:

Physical Examination

Inspection	Shows nothing.
Palpation	May actually reveal a step-off between the spinous processes of the slipped vertebra and the adjacent vertebra below. There may or may not be tenderness.
Range of Motion	Usually normal.
Orthopaedic and Neurologic Tests	Most will be normal. However, there are almost always findings of hamstring tightness. The hamstrings are the group of big muscles on the back of the thigh. They begin on the back of the pelvis above the hip joint and end just below the knee joint. This means that the hamstrings span two joints. As spondylolisthesis occurs, the forward slipping of the lower lumbar vertebra results in a change in posture: Lordosis increases and the pelvis tilts forward. (**Fig. 4–14**) To maintain balance, the hips and knees bend a little. (We say they flex.) This shortens the distance the hamstrings have to span, and they tighten or shrink.

Tests You Might Have	What They Might Show
Lumbar Spine X-rays	Lumbar spine x-rays will be dramatic and absolutely diagnostic: The side view will show the spondylolisthesis, (**Fig. 4–15**) and the oblique views will show the bilateral spondylolysis.
MRI Scan and CAT Scan Studies	Again, these tests will show the changes, but as before, they are usually not needed.
EMGs and NCTs	Not needed, unless the patient has some neurologic symptoms or changes, which are fairly unusual.

Figure 4-14

Spondylolisthesis Causing Tight Hamstrings

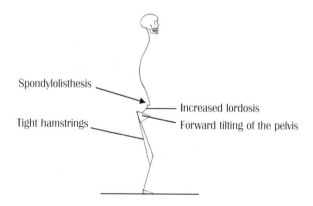

Spondylolisthesis

Tight hamstrings

Increased lordosis

Forward tilting of the pelvis

Figure 4-15

X-ray Showing Spondylolisthesis

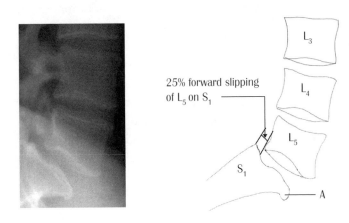

25% forward slipping of L_5 on S_1

L_3

L_4

L_5

S_1

A

X-ray Vision

Notice that the anterior superior (front upper) corner of the first sacral vertebra **(A)** is rounded off and pushed downward. That's because the loose, unconnected body of the fifth lumbar vertebra constantly pushed against it each of the tens of thousands of times this patient flexed (bent forward) over the years. This constant, repetitive pressure against that edge of the first sacral vertebra did two things: It wore it down, and it caused that edge to remodel, or reshape, as a response.

DEGENERATIVE SPONDYLOLISTHESIS

Degenerative spondylolisthesis is actually a special form of degenerative arthritis of the spine, which you learned about earlier. Unlike the spondylolisthesis that's just been discussed, this condition arises as a result of severe degeneration of a pair of facet joints of one vertebra, which causes the upper half of the facet to slide in relation to the lower half. At the same time, the intervertebral disc at that level will have also degenerated, and the anterior and posterior longitudinal ligaments surrounding that disc will have stretched. Note that I've made no mention of spondylolysis. That's because it doesn't occur in this special condition.

The symptoms associated with degenerative spondylolisthesis will be a combination of those related to arthritis and those related to nerve root irritation. There will often be impingement of the bony structures or disc against a nerve root exiting on one side, the nerve roots exiting on both sides, and/or the thecal sac covering the nerve roots in the spinal canal.

Take a look at our simplified chart:

PHYSICAL EXAMINATION

Inspection	Usually shows loss of lordosis.
Palpation	Reveals diffuse tenderness.
Range of Motion	Will show painful, limited motion often with absence of reversal of lordosis on forward flexion.
Orthopaedic and Neurologic Tests	Frequently, will show signs of nerve root irritation including sensory changes or motor weakness or diminution of reflexes along with signs of nerve root tightness.

TESTS YOU MIGHT HAVE	**WHAT THEY MIGHT SHOW**
Lumbar Spine X-rays	Lumbar spine x-rays will clearly show degenerative spondylolisthesis on the lateral (side) and oblique (partially turned) views. (**Fig. 4–16**)
Lumbar Myelogram	Will show whether there is compression of the thecal sac and the extent of any kinking of the thecal sac at that area. (**Fig. 4–17**)
MRI Scan and CAT Scan Studies	Will confirm the diagnosis, while also showing if a nerve root or roots and/or the thecal sac have been impinged upon or indented.
EMGs and NCTs	Can show evidence of nerve root irritation if the nerve roots have been either stretched or impinged upon by the bone spurs and/or the disc.

Figure 4-16

X-ray Showing Degenerative Spondylolisthesis

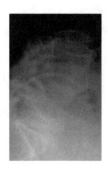

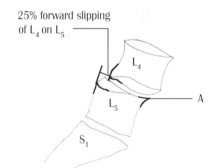

25% forward slipping of L_4 on L_5

L_4

L_5

S_1

A

X-ray Vision

The x-ray on page 107 shows a degenerative spondylolisthesis that occurred one level higher than the spondylolisthesis we saw in Figure 4–15. Since this x-ray shows a degenerative condition, notice that the anterior superior (front upper) corner of the fifth lumbar vertebra **(A)** did not round off or remodel. That's because the pars interarticularis (the "neck" of the Scottie dog) remained intact. As a result, the front and back halves of the fourth lumbar vertebra remained solidly connected to each other. Hence, when this patient flexed (bent forward), the vertebral body was not unstable and could not exert extra pressure at **(A)**.

Figure 4-17

Myelogram Showing Degenerative Spondylolisthesis

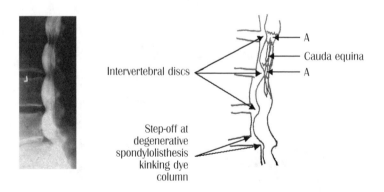

X-ray Vision

This patient also has spinal stenosis. That's why the column of dye has the wavy appearance to it as it gets indented, in turn, by each

intervertebral disc that is protruding posteriorly. Also at each indentation, the column of dye is much darker and less white **(A)** because
the constriction limits the amount of dye which can get through. Notice how the degenerative spondylolisthesis has created a step-off
that constricts and kinks the nerve roots. You can also see the cauda
equina.

The x-ray technician put an "L" marker on the film cassette which appears backwards on the film. But there is no left or right on a lateral
(side) view.

TRANSITIONAL VERTEBRAE

You learned in chapter 1 that there are five lumbar vertebrae, as well as
five sacral vertebrae that are fused together to make a firm, bony anchor for the spine. (**Fig. 4–18**)

Figure 4-18

Sacrum

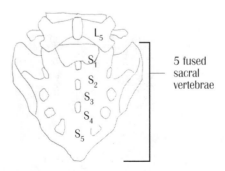

That's the way it's supposed to work, and in fact it does work that way most of the time. But not always. Sometimes, while a fetus is being formed, something happens during the process called segmentation, when the individual vertebrae are forming. What happens is that the fifth lumbar vertebra (known as L_5 in medical shorthand), which sits directly above the sacrum, doesn't quite fully separate from the sacrum. When this occurs, the transverse process of the fifth lumbar vertebra—which is just a little nubbin—takes on the appearance of a large sacral transverse process and may actually fuse with the transverse process of the sacrum.

If this takes place on only one side of the vertebra, it's called hemisacralization of the fifth lumbar vertebra. (**Fig. 4–19**) If it happens with both transverse processes of L_5, we call it sacralization of L_5. (**Fig. 4–20**) The enlarged transverse process or processes will frequently act as a tether, preventing the nice free motion that normally can occur at L_5. The transverse process may also create a false joint with the adjacent ilium, and this can result in mechanical rubbing of the two bones.

Figure 4-19

X-ray Showing Hemisacralization

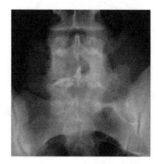

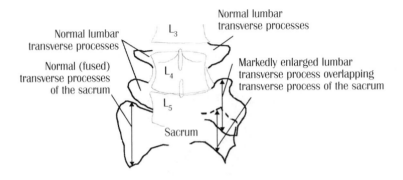

Normal lumbar
transverse processes

Normal lumbar
transverse processes

L₃

Normal (fused)
transverse processes
of the sacrum

L₄

Markedly enlarged lumbar
transverse process overlapping
transverse process of the sacrum

L₅

Sacrum

X-ray Vision

If you put a piece of paper over the right half of the x-ray on page 110, the left half shows two normal lumbar transverse processes plus the fused transverse processes of the sacrum. Now if you shift the paper and cover the left side of the x-ray, the right half appears to show just one normal lumbar transverse process plus the sacrum.

The fifth lumbar vertebra appears to extend below the top of the sacrum. It's just an optical illusion because the x-ray is a two-dimensional representation that "flattens" the lumbar lordosis, causing one vertebra to be superimposed on the next.

There can be another error of segmentation. The first sacral vertebra, S₁, may partially or completely segment, and thus be separate from the second sacral vertebra, S₂. This is called lumbarization of the first sacral vertebra. (**Fig. 4–21**) There may even be an intervertebral disc between S₁ and S₂. Not only will there be some slight mobility of a structure that's supposed to be solid and rigid, but there will also be a smaller mass of solid, immobile sacrum acting as the base of the spine.

Figure 4-20

Front-View X-ray Showing Complete Sacralization

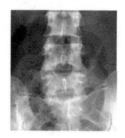

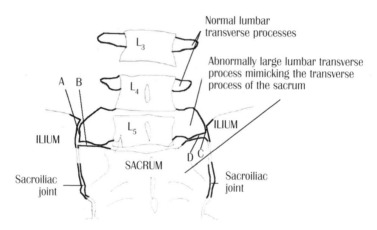

X-ray Vision

On this x-ray, we see four false joints that normally don't exist. The huge abnormal transverse processes of the fifth lumbar vertebra make false joints with the left and right ilium bone at **(A)** and **(C),** and with the top of the normal fused transverse processes of the sacrum on the left and right at **(B)** and **(D)**. These false joints are actually formed just like real joints, and they have cartilage covering their surfaces. There would be no cartilage in these specific areas if the fifth lumbar transverse processes were of normal size.

Figure 4-21

Front-View X-ray Showing Lumbarization

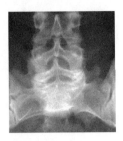

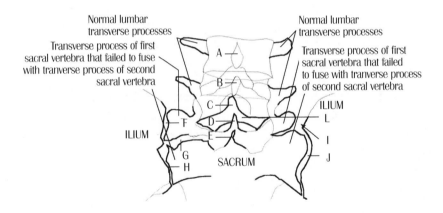

Normal lumbar transverse processes

Transverse process of first sacral vertebra that failed to fuse with tranverse process of second sacral vertebra

ILIUM

Normal lumbar transverse processes

Transverse process of first sacral vertebra that failed to fuse with tranverse process of second sacral vertebra

ILIUM

A

B

C

F D

E

G

H

SACRUM

ILIUM

L

I

J

X-ray Vision

How did I know that this x-ray really shows an abnormal first sacral vertebra with its own lumbar-appearing discreet lamina and transverse processes? I cheated! There are other x-rays of this patient that show that there are 12 normal thoracic vertebrae with 12 pairs of ribs, and under them are five normal lumbar vertebrae, and then there is this sacral abnormality.

(A) and **(B)** are the spinous processes of the fourth and fifth lumbar vertebrae; **(C)**, **(D)**, and **(E)** are the spinous processes of the first three sacral vertebrae.

Notice how the laminae of the first sacral vertebra **(L)** have failed to fuse with the laminae of the second sacral vertebra and thus look just like the laminae of a lumbar vertebra.

There is a sacroiliac joint between the transverse process of the first sacral vertebra and the ilium on the left side **(F)**, but because that transverse process is not fused to the transverse process below it, it will move abnormally and may cause severe pain. There is also a false joint **(G)** between the transverse processes on the left side of the first and second sacral vertebrae.

There is a normal sacroiliac joint on the left side **(H)**, and on the right side **(J)** where there is no false joint between it and the ilium **(I)**.

Bending, twisting, lifting, and the like can all result in irritation of a transitional vertebra, causing sudden sharp lumbosacral pain. This may be quite localized to the lumbosacral junction. Sometimes, however, it may be accompanied by radiating leg pain from the mechanical rubbing of an enlarged transverse process against the ilium.

Here's the chart for this condition:

PHYSICAL EXAMINATION

Inspection	May show loss of lordosis and/or a sciatic shift.
Palpation	Will often reveal exquisite point tenderness directly over the enlarged transverse process(es) of a hemisacralized or sacralized L_5. There may also be spasm.

Range of Motion	May reveal limitation of motion due to pain, spasm, or both.

Tests You Might Have	**What They Might Show**
Lumbar Spine X-rays	The front view x-ray of the lumbar spine allows an instant diagnosis: The hemisacralization or complete sacralization of L_5 or the lumbarization of S_1 can be seen quite clearly.
MRI Scan and CAT Scan Studies	Not needed since this is purely a mechanical problem.
EMGs and NCTs	Rarely necessary.

Now you've learned about the common causes of acute and chronic back pain and how they're diagnosed. Ready to learn how to treat them? Turn the page!

Chapter Five

HOW WE TREAT THE INJURED BACK
THE TECHNIQUES THAT WE USE

Many of the acute injuries and problems and chronic conditions that cause back pain can be treated without resorting to surgery. Unfortunately, nonoperative treatment won't always be successful, and sometimes surgery is needed to correct a problem. In fact, it's important to keep in mind that while certain problems never, ever need surgery, other conditions *always* do.

Before you learn how different problems are treated, you need to learn about the various treatment methods that are used. That way, you'll understand why they are used and how they help the back to heal.

Physical Therapy

Physical therapy is just what the name implies: a type of treatment that is used externally and involves a variety of mechanical means to try to heal structures deep inside the body. A physical therapist has had at least two to four years of college training, plus training in an accredited physical therapy program. Physical therapists use a variety of techniques to treat painful conditions of the muscles, ligaments, tendons, bones, and joints. These techniques are divided into several categories: modalities, massage, stretching exercises, and strengthening exercises.

MODALITIES

Heat

Heat is the most common modality used, and it comes in two varieties: dry and moist. Dry heat—the kind you get from an electric heating pad or a hot-water bottle—is actually fairly useless because it really doesn't penetrate more than three millimeters below the surface of the skin.

Junior Doctor's Merit Badge Checkpoint

Keep in mind that a average adult has 0.5 to 2 inches (1.25 to 5 centimeters) of fatty tissue below the skin's surface in the lumbar region. Overweight people may have as much as 4 inches (10 centimeters) of fat below the skin surface. Underneath whatever fat is present lies a sheath of gristle tissue that surrounds all the paraspinal muscles to contain them, and that attaches to the very top edge of the spinous processes (the chimneys of our vertebral houses). This gristle tissue, called the **lumbodorsal fascia**, separates the fat from the muscle. **(Fig. 5-1)**

Moist heat, however, can be of some benefit. Fat is a good insulator and thus will tend to keep heat—especially dry heat—away from the muscles. But moist heat penetrates up to about an inch (2 centimeters) below the surface of the skin. So in a person of average or slim build, moist heat will penetrate to the superficial part of the paraspinal muscles. Moist heat relaxes muscles by making the tiny blood vessels, the **capillaries**, dilate. When they do, more blood flows through them, and, since blood has a temperature of 98.6 degrees F (37 degrees C), it heats up the muscle tissue. Increased blood flow helps alleviate spasm or tightness, and that, in turn, helps relieve pain.

Figure 5 - 1

Cross-section MRI Showing the Layers of the Back

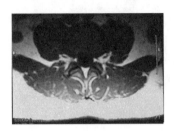

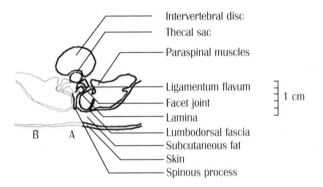

Intervertebral disc
Thecal sac
Paraspinal muscles

Ligamentum flavum
Facet joint   1 cm
Lamina
B   A   Lumbodorsal fascia
Subcutaneous fat
Skin
Spinous process

X-ray Vision

Notice that there is a centimeter scale on the right side of the MRI film. This allows us to see exactly the size of various structures. For instance, on this patient, the skin is just 2 millimeters thick, while the subcutaneous fat is 2 centimeters thick at the very center **(A)**, and becomes over 4 centimeters thick just 7 centimeters farther to the side **(B)**. The thecal sac is 1.5 centimeters in diameter, and it is about 8 centimeters below the surface of the skin. The paraspinal muscles are about 3 centimeters thick, and they are 3 to 8 centimeters beneath the skin surface. Now you see why dry heat doesn't work!

To Make a Moist Hot Compress

Take a towel, soak it in hot water, wring it out, fold it over on itself, and place it on the sore part of your back as you lie on your stomach. Place a hot-water bottle on top of the moist, hot towel, and cover the hot-water bottle and towel with waxed paper. Over the waxed paper place a second folded, dry towel or a small folded blanket. These layers will keep the heat from escaping, and the heat will last for thirty to forty-five minutes.

ICE

Ice is rarely used to treat back pain. It *is* quite effective in the immediate treatment of sports injuries, such as ankle and knee sprains and the like, where swelling has occurred. Whereas heat helps capillaries dilate and increases blood flow, ice constricts capillaries, reduces blood flow, lowers the tissue temperature, and thus helps reduce swelling. Ice penetrates deeper than moist heat (think of the conditions people suffer from due to prolonged outdoor exposure to cold). But back injuries and conditions causing back pain don't tend to cause swelling of the paraspinal muscles, so it doesn't really make sense to treat back pain with ice.

ULTRASOUND

Ultrasound involves the use of high-frequency sound waves; in fact, they're so high frequency that you don't hear them. Ultrasound is a wonderful deep-heating modality because it can penetrate up to 7 inches (17.5 centimeters) below the surface of the skin. This means ultrasound can penetrate all the way through to the deepest paraspinal muscles in an average-sized adult. It's great for increasing the **distensibility** (stretchability) of muscle tissue. Like moist heat, ultrasound makes capillaries dilate, improves blood flow, reduces spasm and stiffness, and alleviates pain. It can be of considerable help in improving segmental spinal range of motion—that's the motion between pairs of vertebrae that allows you to bend and twist normally—as well as sciatic shift. As motion improves, the ultrasound can be reduced and then eliminated.

Acute and chronic back problems often benefit from the use of ultrasound, because it provides pain relief and increased flexibility that allows the physical therapist to utilize various stretches, massages, and exercises with the patient. Ultrasound is never used if there is any question of infection or tumor, in children or adolescents who are still growing (because it can heat up the growth plates of bones and damage them), or in pregnant women. It should also be used very judiciously in patients who have already had back surgery because it can damage their scar tissue.

> **Therapeutic ultrasound**, the kind we've been discussing here, is designed to generate heat. That's what gives it its healing properties. But excess heat can harm a fetus. We say it is **teratogenic**. **Diagnostic ultrasound**, the ultrasound that's used to see the fetus in the uterus in pregnant women, is much less intense and generates no heat. That's why it's safe to use during pregnancy.

HIGH-VOLTAGE GALVANIC STIMULATION

High-voltage galvanic stimulation is a type of electrical stimulation; it's also called **microdyne**. Now, this is not the kind of electric shock treatment that's accompanied by someone saying, "You *will* tell us everything we want to know." Additionally, it is not the kind of electric shock treatment that's used to treat certain mental illnesses. Instead, this electric shock is delivered to the skin and transmitted to the underlying muscle. Strangely, by making the muscles contract and relax repeatedly, high-voltage galvanic stimulation is thought to reduce the ability of the muscle to contract. (It kind of fatigues the muscle.) So it's best used only during the early stages of acute lower back pain when there may be muscle spasm, and, in the case of a sprain/strain, microscopic amounts of blood leaking into the muscle (which I'll talk about later on, in chapter 6). There isn't a tremendous amount of scientific evidence indicating that it really works, but some studies show that it does.

MASSAGE

Massage is pretty much just what you'd think it is: a technique involving kneading all the back muscles with the therapist's hands and fingers in an attempt to break up tension and spasm and to relax the muscles. A variation is ice massage, but this is done only rarely for back pain.

DEEP FRICTION MASSAGE

Also called **transverse friction massage**, deep friction massage is a massage technique in which the therapist applies very strong pressure transverse to the direction of the muscle fibers. It is done with the therapist's fingers and is applied directly to a specific tender spot. When done properly, the technique does not cause pain; if pain occurs, it is because either the technique is being incorrectly performed, or an excessive amount of pressure is being applied. In fact, when correctly done, deep friction massage tends to make the area numb briefly. It can significantly ease pain in so-called trigger areas, and it relieves highly localized back pain. Some researchers have suggested that it may help promote the early stages of tissue repair after an injury. I'll discuss that in more detail later on in this chapter.

STRETCHING EXERCISES

You learned in the section on spondylolisthesis in chapter 4 that hamstring tightness is often seen in that condition. In fact, not only does hamstring tightness often *lead* to back pain by reducing mobility, but it also seems to be found frequently in people who have back pain.

Remember: The hamstrings span two joints. They start from the pelvic bones, go across the back of the hip joint, go all the way down the back of the thighbone (the femur), cross the back of the knee joint, and attach to the upper part of the back of the shinbone (the tibia).

The normal back is a highly mobile structure: We can bend forward and touch our toes, bend sideways at the waist, and so forth. Tight hamstrings keep us from doing these things. Stretching exercises help overcome and correct this, restoring flexibility to the spine and reducing pain. When done regularly, stretching exercises may also help prevent recurrences of episodes of back pain. I'll discuss stretching exercises in detail later in this chapter.

STRENGTHENING EXERCISES

Don't think of pumping iron at the gym when you read about strengthening exercises. You're not trying to build up your arm and leg muscles; instead, you're working on the muscles of the back and abdomen.

Remember: The abdominal muscles allow you to bend forward, or flex.

There are three main types of strengthening exercises. Some therapists use one type exclusively; some incorporate both types in a rehabilitation program, depending on their training as well as the type of condition being treated.

MCKENZIE EXTENSION EXERCISES

McKenzie extension exercises were developed by a New Zealand physical therapist named Robin McKenzie. They involve a series of extension exercises in which the posterior paraspinal muscles are strengthened. Remember how I showed you that a herniated disc extrudes posteriorly, or backward? This almost always occurs because of something that happened while the patient was flexing, or bending forward. So, McKenzie believes, reducing flexion and increasing extension takes the pressure off the posterior part of the disc. If the McKenzie program is successful, the radiating leg pain should resolve and the pain should localize (or, in McKenzie's terms, centralize) in the low back, and eventually disappear.

FLEXION EXERCISES

Flexion exercises are just the opposite of McKenzie extension exercises, and they are used to strengthen the abdominal muscles. You learned in the section on degenerative arthritis in chapter 4 that there's a force of fifteen pounds per square inch across a lower lumbar disc for each pound that's lifted with the arm outstretched. Well, if you suck in your belly while you're lifting something, you actually reduce the force across the discs because you've turned your entire abdominal cavity into a hydraulic pump. We say in medical terms that tightening the abdominal muscles during lifting or carrying unloads the lumbar spine. Flexion exercises help improve this ability, and thus they help relieve some kinds of back pain.

DYNAMIC STABILIZATION EXERCISES

Dynamic stabilization exercises are a third type of strengthening exercises and are based on the concept that the back has a position it likes because it doesn't hurt in that position. So if you have back pain as a result of some condition or problem, the therapist tries to find the particular erect position of the spine that's either pain-free or the least painful. (It's called the neutral position.) The therapist then has the patient exercise the back muscles in that position to train them to be the strongest in that position so that pain will be relieved. These are vigorous exercises and are not suitable for all causes of back pain.

On Your Own

AEROBIC EXERCISES

Exercises that increase the heart rate and the breathing rate are called **aerobic exercises**. They can be either low impact, meaning they don't put any severe stress on the joints, or they can be high impact—think of the drill-sergeant-like instructor who has you kicking, jumping, lunging, stepping up and down, and so on. High-impact aerobics are not done for the back, but low-impact aerobic exercises can be quite helpful. There are three that work best:

WATER (POOL) EXERCISES

Water (pool) exercises have the great advantage that, because the body is weightless in the water, it's easier for you to move. Thus increased motion can be regained with less or no pain, while the decreased stress of doing exercises in the water helps improve conditioning.

WALKING

Walking is another exercise that does not place stress on the back, but it does help improve its strength and your overall conditioning.

EXERCISE BICYCLING

Exercise bicycling on a stationary bike keeps the spine in proper posture, allows the muscles to strengthen, may be less stressful on the back than walking, and also is good for conditioning.

HOME EXERCISES

If you suffer from back pain, one of the most important things you can do is a series of simple exercises at home. You don't need any equipment, the exercises are really easy, and they can be of great help in relieving pain and stiffness. Certain moves should not be done if your pain is due to certain specific problems. In the subsequent sections of this chapter, I'll tell you which exercises to avoid when. Here I'm going to explain to you how to do each of them. Of course, these should only be used after your back problem has been diagnosed by your doctor.

PRONE EXTENSION

Prone extension is the easiest of all.

✦ Lie down on the floor on your stomach with your elbows bent and your hands next to your shoulders. (**Fig. 5–2A**) If your back pain is on just one side, shift your hips toward the other side a bit.

✦ Push down on your hands and slowly straighten your elbows and look straight ahead. Keep your pelvis and legs relaxed, and hold this position for three to five seconds. (**Fig. 5–2B**)

✦ Then slowly return to the resting position.

✦ You can repeat this exercise twenty to thirty times, and you can do it two, three, or four times a day.

STANDING EXTENSION

Standing extension is a variation on prone extension.

✦ Stand with your feet just slightly apart. Put your hands at the small of the back with the fingers pointing toward each other. (**Fig. 5–3A**)

✦ Bend back slowly and hold for several seconds, then slowly return to the resting position. (**Fig. 5–3B**)

✦ You can repeat this exercise twenty to thirty times, and you can do it two, three, or four times a day.

Figure 5-2

Prone Extension

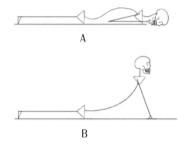

A

B

Figure 5-3

Standing Extension

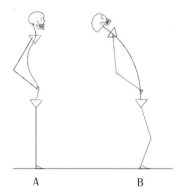

A   B

SITTING FLEXION

Sitting flexion will do the opposite of the extension exercises above.

+ Sit on a firm chair or stool with your legs apart (forming a V) and your hands resting on your knees. (**Fig. 5–4A**)

+ Bend forward slowly at the waist, touching the floor with your hands. Hold this position for three to five seconds and then slowly return to the sitting position. (**Fig. 5–4B**)

+ You can repeat this exercise twenty to thirty times, and you can do it two, three, or four times a day. As you develop flexibility and your pain decreases, you can gain more flexion bending forward by holding on to your ankles and pulling yourself into more flexion. (**Fig. 5–4C**)

Figure 5-4

Sitting Flexion

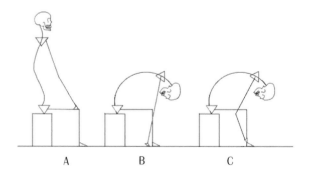

A   B   C

SUPINE FLEXION

Supine flexion is a variation of the previous exercise.

✦ Lie on the floor on your back with your hands at your sides and your knees bent to a comfortable degree. As you do this exercise, *keep your knees bent at all times and do not straighten your legs.* (**Fig. 5–5A**)

✦ Hold on to your knees with your hands (**Fig. 5–5B**) and pull your knees toward your chest as far as you can. (**Fig. 5–5C**)

✦ Hold this position for three to five seconds and then slowly return to the resting position. *Keep the back of your head on the floor and do not raise it while you do this exercise.*

✦ You can repeat this exercise twenty to thirty times, and you can do it two, three, or four times a day.

Figure 5-5

Supine Flexion

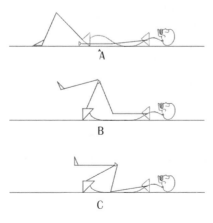

Sitting Flexion to Extension

Sitting flexion to extension is very easy to do.

- ✦ Sit on a firm chair or stool with your legs in front of you.

- ✦ Sit in a very slouched position for several seconds. (No, I haven't lost my mind!) **(Fig. 5–6A)** Then slowly straighten up and make your back as extended as possible—the other extreme— with a nice hollow in it. **(Fig. 5–6B)**

- ✦ Hold this for three to five seconds and then return to the first position. It's important to do this slowly and smoothly, without any jerky movements.

- ✦ You can repeat this exercise twenty to thirty times, and you can do it two, three, or four times a day. This exercise is really good if you have back pain and must continue to work at a job that involves prolonged sitting.

Figure 5-6

Sitting Flexion to Extension

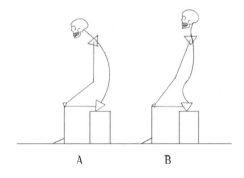

A　　　　B

SACROILIAC STRETCHING

Sacroiliac stretching involves two easily done exercises that help open up the irritated sacroiliac joint.

✦ For the first exercise, lie on the floor on your back with your legs out straight. Ideally you should have someone push down on the bony bump (called the anterior superior iliac spine or ASIS) that's located in line with your belly button but at the front side of the pelvic bone (the ilium). It's just above each hip joint. (**Fig. 5–7**) You want the one on the same side as the sore sacroiliac joint (which, of course, is on the back side of the pelvis). (**Fig. 5–8A**)

✦ While the ASIS is held still or is being pushed down, either swing that leg with the knee straight across the other leg as far as possible and hold for about five seconds (**Fig. 5–8B**) or bend the knee of that leg and try to get that knee across the other leg down toward the floor for about five seconds. (**Fig. 5–8C**)

Figure 5-7

Anterior Superior Iliac Spine

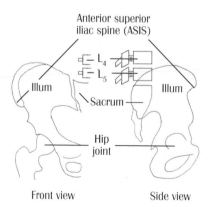

Front view   Side view

✦ It isn't easy, but with practice, you'll get the hang of it. Repeat it ten to twenty times, and do it two or three times daily.

The second exercise is done on either a bed or a sofa.

✦ This time, lie on your stomach with the half of your pelvis that includes the sore sacroiliac joint out in space beyond the edge of the bed or sofa. **(Fig. 5–9A)**

✦ Keeping the good leg firmly pressed into the bed or sofa, bend the knee on the sore side, trying to bring the knee down to the floor. **(Fig. 5–9B)**

✦ Hold for about five seconds, repeat ten to twenty times, and do this two to three times daily.

Figure 5-8

Sacroiliac Stretching

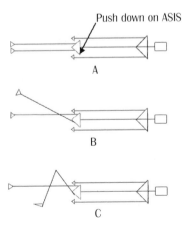

Prone Sacroiliac Stretching

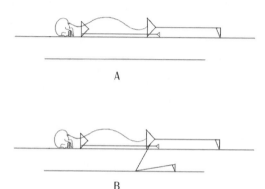

A

B

Braces and Belts

Did you ever go to a big home improvement store, a nursing home, or somewhere else where lifting and carrying is done, and see workers wearing back supports, usually with straps that go over their shoulders? Well, guess what? Those things are pretty much useless. A number of large studies have shown that they really don't *prevent* low back injuries. The best thing they do is serve as a reminder to the wearer to lift and carry properly.

Some devices, however, do have limited benefit for patients whose back pain comes from certain conditions. An irritated sacroiliac joint—caused by a sprain of the sacroiliac ligaments—may benefit from a **sacroiliac belt**. It's just what it sounds like: a wide, flat, mildly elastic belt that goes around the body at the upper part of the ilium bones and helps compress them against the sacrum. That compression can help keep the sacroiliac joints from shifting or moving (remember, the amount of motion is extremely small), and that reduces pain.

There are certain **rigid back braces** that can be helpful in reducing back pain, especially for mechanical conditions such as spondylolysis, spondylolisthesis, facet joint irritation, degenerative arthritis, and the like, or in the treatment of compression fractures. These braces must be prescribed by a physician, and they are fabricated specifically for one patient based on his or her measurements. Although these braces will not prevent 100 percent of motion in the lower lumbar spine, they do reduce and restrict motion enough to help relieve pain by decreasing the motions that cause it. There are many types and designs; some are rigid plastic shells, others are steel covered with leather, and still others are aluminum.

Medication

There are three types of medicines that can be helpful in the treatment of back pain: pain medicines (which we call analgesics), arthritis medicines, and muscle relaxants.

ANALGESICS

Let's take a look at what's really in some of the most popular over-the-counter **pain relievers**.

BRAND NAME	ACTIVE INGREDIENT AND WHAT IT DOES
Aspirin	**Acetylsalicylic acid** (the chemical name for aspirin)—relieves pain and has an anti-inflammatory ability.
Tylenol	**Acetaminophen** (the part of the aspirin molecule that relieves pain)—no anti-inflammatory ability.
Excedrin	Contains both aspirin and acetaminophen—so it both relieves pain and decreases inflammation.

Prescription analgesics are narcotics or narcotic-like medicines. This means that they are often habit forming—you may become addicted to them. Some of them, in fact, are addicting within *as little as one to three weeks*. My opinion is that they rarely have a place in the treatment of acute lower back pain regardless of its cause. There's no question that they may give excellent pain relief, but no pain medicine relieves the *cause* of pain—the medicine only relieves the *symptom*, pain itself.

ARTHRITIS MEDICINES

Arthritis medicines are actually **NSAIDs**, or nonsteroidal anti-inflammatory drugs. This means that they reduce inflammation but do not contain any cortisone (steroid). Some can be purchased either as over-the-counter (OTC) medicines in a lower strength or in a prescription form in full strength. Others can only be obtained by prescription.

Here are some of the popular OTC NSAIDs—all of them will help reduce inflammation and pain. You may have to try each of these because some patients may develop stomach upset with one and not with another.

BRAND NAME	ACTIVE INGREDIENT
Advil	Ibuprofen
Aleve	Naproxen
Orudis	Ketoprofen

The prescription-strength NSAIDs work via a number of different mechanisms, which is why one may worth better for you than another. Here's a partial list, with the generic name given in parentheses:

+ Celebrex (celecoxib)
+ Clinoril (sulindac)
+ Daypro (oxaprozin)

- Indocin (indomethacin)
- Lodine (etodolac)
- Nalfon (fenoprofen)
- Orudis, Oruvail (ketoprofen)
- Relafen (nabumetone)
- Tolectin (tolmetin)
- Toradol (ketorolac)
- Vioxx (rofecoxib)
- Voltaren (diclofenac)

By reducing inflammation, they can attack the cause of many types of back pain, including sprains, strains, irritation of facet and sacroiliac joints, degenerative arthritis, and more. They won't cure arthritis, but they can greatly relieve the symptoms it causes. Of course, they all have side effects, and naturally, care must be taken in using them so that you don't trade in one problem (back pain) for another, such as stomach bleeding.

MUSCLE RELAXANTS

Muscle relaxants have a limited, but sometimes effective, role. They may have some ability to relieve spasm, but they rarely can make spasm disappear in a flash. For muscle relaxants to be effective, several things have to happen. First—and this isn't as dumb as it sounds—there has to be spasm.

 Remember: Spasm is frequently overdiagnosed during the inspection and palpation parts of a physical examination.

If the examining doctor thinks that there's spasm present but there isn't, then a muscle relaxant won't do anything. Second, spasm won't go away unless we can correct the underlying problem that caused it to occur. Remember that spasm is a protective mechanism of the body to prevent motion of an area that's injured, so as we fix the injured part, we give the muscle relaxant the ability to do its job. Unfortunately, muscle relaxants don't just relax the paraspinal muscles at the area of injury; they can have similar effects throughout the body—which means your whole body might feel a little bit unsteady, and you may get very sleepy after taking a muscle relaxant.

Muscle relaxants are all prescription medicines. Here's a partial list of them:

+ Flexeril (cyclobenzaprine)

+ Norflex (orphenadrine)

+ Norgesic Forte (ophenadrine + aspirin + caffeine)

+ Parafon Forte (chlorzoxazone)

+ Robaxin (methocarbamol)

+ Skelaxin (metaxalone)

+ Soma (carisoprodol)

+ Valium (diazepam)

+ Zanaflex (tizanidine)

Injections

Some anaesthesiologists have subspecialized and offer pain management in which they treat certain back problems with special injections. Although this is usually done for the patient with chronic complaints of pain from such conditions as failed back surgery, degenerative arthritis, and degenerative disc disease, there are some acute conditions, such as a flare-up or facet joint pain or of sacroiliac irritation, for which injections may be helpful.

Surgery

What I've discussed so far in this chapter have been what are collectively called nonoperative forms of treatment. But as I said at the beginning of this chapter, some back problems simply won't get better unless they are treated surgically. I'm not going to make you a surgeon in one easy lesson, but I do want you to know what's generally involved when surgery is performed. Here are five common procedures.

LUMBAR LAMINECTOMY

For more than fifty years, lumbar laminectomy was the standard operation for removing a herniated disc. Lamina, you'll recall, is the Latin word for roof. But tomos is the *Greek* word for cut, so doctors can demonstrate their great classical knowledge by combining Latin and Greek in one word. In this operation, a longitudinal incision is centered over the spinous processes and made through the skin down the very center of the back, the fatty tissue under the skin (called the **subcutaneous tissue**), and the **lumbodorsal fascia** (the gristle covering under that, which is attached to the tips of the spinous processes). The paraspinal muscles are then peeled off the laminae and ligamentum flavum, and a portion of the laminae plus the connecting ligamentum flavum are removed (that's the laminectomy). The dura and nerve root are gently retracted, and the disc is removed. If the disc exploded through the posterior longitudinal ligament, it will be lying free in the spinal canal. If the posterior longitudinal ligament remained intact, it needs to be cut where it covers the disc so special instruments can be inserted to remove the disc fragments. Then the muscles, lumbodorsal fascia, subcutaneous tissue, and skin are sutured or stapled back together. Often a piece of subcutaneous fatty tissue is snipped off and placed over the hole where the laminae and ligamentum flavum were removed (the laminectomy site) to try to minimize the formation of scar tissue on the dura. The surgery takes about one to two hours, and full recovery usually takes from six to twelve weeks.

Lumbar Microdiscectomy

Lumbar microdiscectomy is a variation on the lumbar laminectomy. A much smaller skin incision is made, only a small area of paraspinal muscle is peeled off the lamina, and an operating microscope or special binoculars attached to the surgeon's glasses are used to magnify the operative field and allow a very minimal amount of lamina to be removed along with the ligamentum flavum. Many doctors feel that because this procedure offers less disruption of the deeper tissues, it may result in less scarring and a quicker recovery. A lumbar microdiscectomy takes about one to two hours, and recovery generally takes four to six weeks.

Automated Percutaneous Lumbar Microdiscectomy

Automated percutaneous lumbar microdiscectomy is a more recent development. A small (0.3 inch or 1 centimeter) skin incision is made off to the side, and a long, fat needle or trochar is inserted through the various layers, eventually penetrating the posterior longitudinal ligament and disc. (This is very similar so far to the technique described in chapter 2 for doing a discogram.) This is all observed on a videofluoroscope, a television x-ray machine. After tests are done to make certain the needle is in the right place, a kind of miniature motorized grinder attached to a vacuum is inserted through the trochar and the disc is ground up and suctioned out. A laser can also be inserted to vaporize the disc fragments. If there is a free fragment of disc that has burst through the posterior longitudinal ligament and is lying free in the spinal canal, it can sometimes be difficult—if not impossible—to remove by this technique. The advantage of this technique is that there's usually a very rapid recovery, often one to two weeks.

Chemonucleolysis

Chemonucleolysis (which means chemically dissolving the nucleus pulposus) was in vogue for a while, but it is now used only rarely. It can be done with the patient awake. As with the technique just described previously, a trochar is inserted from off to the side and advanced into the center of the disc. It *must* be in the center of the disc and not in the annulus fibrosus (you'll see why shortly), and its position is verified with a videofluoroscope. Next, just a few cubic centimeters of an enzyme called chymopapain are injected. Chymopapain comes from the papaya plant and has the ability to dissolve the nucleus pulposus, but it has no effect on the annulus fibrosus. It's the purified, fancy medical form of a popular meat tenderizer you can purchase in the supermarket. Unfortunately, it has some very bad side effects. If it leaks out into the spinal canal (because of a free fragment of disc that burst through the posterior longitudinal ligament, because it escapes as a result of the pressure of injection, or because of incorrect trochar placement), it can cause severe scarring around the dura and nerve roots and result in intractable pain. Even more unfortunately, some people are allergic to chymopapain. Although tests are done ahead of time to look for this, the tests may not be infallible. If a patient who's allergic to chymopapain does have a chemonucleolysis, an anaphylactic reaction may occur. The heart stops, and the patient needs cardiopulmonary resuscitation. Occasionally, CPR may fail, and then the patient dies. On the other hand, if chemonucleolysis does work, recovery may just be a day or two, though some patients experience back spasms for a period of time.

ARTIFICIAL DISC IMPLANTATION

Artificial disc implantation is experimental at the time of this writing. Although early attempts at surgical procedures to insert artificial discs all resulted in failure, recently techniques have been devised that appear to hold promise. Several companies have developed artificial discs that have been implanted and have resulted in virtually pain-free function for up to two years. The surgery involves inserting cobalt-chrome steel plates into the apposing vertebral end plates of the vertebrae on each side of the space from which a degenerated disc has been removed. These metal plates then hold in place a high-density polyethylene cushion that acts as a substitute disc. The time for recovery seems to be quick: Some patients have been back to work in less than a week!

SPINE FUSION

Spine fusion is an operation designed to eliminate the motion between two or more vertebrae. Many different techniques can be used to fuse two or more vertebrae together. The basic assumption with all of them is that pain comes as a result of altered motion. (Something rubs against something else: Bone rubs against bone or nerve root; disc rubs against nerve root; and so forth.) If you take away all motion at that area, you take away pain. Here are some of the techniques.

✦ **Posterior spine fusion.** For many decades, the spine fusion operation consisted of making the same kind of surgical incision as for a laminectomy: going through skin, subcutaneous tissue, lumbodorsal fascia, and detaching the paraspinal muscles from the laminae and spinous processes. Think of the lamina as a peanut butter sandwich: It consists of an **outer cortex**, which is the slice of bread; the **marrow**, which is the peanut butter; and the **inner cortex**, which is the second slice of bread. The outer cortex of the lamina was peeled off as bone shavings— just like whittling wood (and using the same kinds of tools). We say that the lamina was decorticated. Then an incision was made over the ilium bone (hip), and the outer cortex of it was removed. Next, long curls of marrow were taken using those same "wood whittling" tools. These marrow curls, called a bone graft, were then grafted onto, or packed across, the decorticated lamina and everything was sewn back together. The patient was kept on strict bed rest lying down for up to three weeks, then wore a back brace for months. The marrow curls acted like trellises in a garden, and new bone grew through them, fusing one lamina to the next. Unfortunately, this kind of spine fusion had a failure rate—a nonfusion rate—of 7 to 10 percent.

In an attempt to reduce the failure rate as well as to speed up the time for recovery, a number of improvements were made, all of which involved the use of metal devices to give added rigidity along with the fusion I just described. We call these **fusions with instrumentation**.

✦ **Posterior spine fusion with plates.** One of the earliest forms of instrumentation involved attaching a plate with screws to the spinous processes.

✦ **Posterior spine fusion with rods.** Another involved inserting C-shaped hooks, facing away from each other, around the edges of the laminae above and below the level of fusion, and then connecting them with rods that acted like turnbuckles and jacked the laminae apart. The hope with both of these types of fusions was that the rigidity imparted by the plate and screws or by the hooks and rods would literally prevent all motion in the area being fused, thus allowing the marrow curl shavings, the bone graft, a better chance to promote the formation of new bone.

✦ **Posterior spine fusion with pedicle screws.** Because one important source of motion between vertebrae is the facet joints, a fusion technique was developed in which the cartilage lining of the facet joints was removed to expose the marrow, and special screws were inserted that went down through the posterior and anterior facets to compress them tightly together. Considerable surgical skill is required to stay perfectly aligned and thus completely within the rather small facets and pedicles. This is critical to avoid fracturing, or breaking, the facets and to avoid having the ends of the screws project and penetrate adjacent structures such as the nerve root. (**Fig. 5–10**)

✦ **Interbody fusion with metal cage.** In recent years, one newer form of instrumentation involved removing the disc completely and inserting a metal cage in the space between the vertebral bodies. The cage was filled either with bone or with material that helps promote bone growth. Believe it or not, the cage could be inserted from the posterior side of the vertebra, going down between the laminae.

Figure 5-10

Pedicle Screw

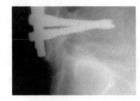

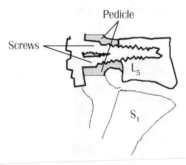

X-ray Vision

The pedicle isn't as thick as it looks on this x-ray. The x-ray beam didn't go precisely perpendicular to the vertebra, causing a kind of magnification distortion. Notice how the screw goes into the vertebral body as well so that it will be solidly anchored.

✦ **Combined anterior interbody and posterior fusion.** A different
approach, literally, was to operate on the spine from the front—
by going through the abdominal cavity. This requires exception-
ally meticulous technique and involves a general surgeon who
must open the abdominal cavity, retract the intestines, and keep
the aorta and its major arteries and the vena cava and its major
veins all out of the way. The orthopaedic surgeon then removes
the *anterior* longitudinal ligament, removes the entire disc from
the front, and then inserts in place of the disc either a wedge-
shaped piece of bone (which was removed from the ilium) or a
metal cage filled with bone. Then the entire wound is repaired
and closed, the patient is often turned over, and a posterior instru-
mented fusion is also performed. (**Fig. 5–11**)

Not surprisingly, patients frequently had a very slow recovery,
and a significant number continued to have chronic pain.

Figure 5-11

Combined Anterior and Posterior Fusion

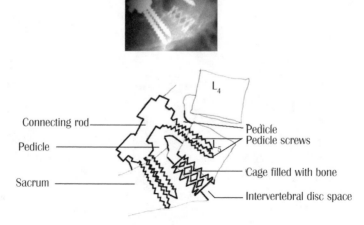

Connecting rod

Pedicle

Sacrum

L₄

L₅

Pedicle
Pedicle screws

Cage filled with bone

Intervertebral disc space

X-ray Vision

On the x-ray on page 144, the bone that's placed inside the cage that is inserted anteriorly in the intervertebral disc space will eventually **fuse**, or unite, with the lower part of the fifth lumbar vertebra and the upper part of the first sacral vertebra. This is called the **anterior column**. There are actually two rods, one to each side of the spinous processes, but they are superimposed on the x-ray. These rods will make the posterior half of the vertebra, called the **posterior column**, rigid as well. In addition, the rods will prevent the fifth lumbar and first sacral vertebrae from coming closer together—a condition called **settling**—during the time it takes for the fusion to become solid.

Now you've seen that there is a broad spectrum of treatment options available to your doctor. These range from very simple, easily performed home exercises to complex, highly technical surgeries. Learning the reasons why various forms of treatment may be helpful for your back pain will make you the darling of your doctor: Not only will you be well informed, but you'll also have wonderful insight into the nature of your problem. There's nothing a doctor enjoys more than a patient who understands what the doctor is talking about!

Chapter Six

Putting It All Together

At last! You've learned how back injuries occur. You've learned the parts of the back that can be injured. You've learned how to diagnose those injuries. You've learned the tests to help confirm your diagnosis. And you've learned the various types of treatment that are available. Now it's time to put all of this together and to learn how to outwit, or treat, your back pain.

Sprains and Strains

The treatment of a sprain/strain of the low back is simple once you understand a little bit of what the body does to heal an injury; this is called the **physiology of healing**.

Remember: The injury in a low back sprain/strain involves microscopic stretching of paraspinal muscles and ligaments, with tearing of individual muscle cells and capillaries, and spilling out of individual blood cells and the contents of the individual muscle cells. This creates intense muscle contraction, or spasm.

The body's reaction to a sprain or strain is an immediate attempt to repair the damage. Such repair occurs in three stages: inflammatory, proliferative, and remodeling.

INFLAMMATORY STAGE

In the **inflammatory stage**, which occurs first:

✦ The body sends specialized white blood cells to the area to begin to clean up all that debris between and around cells and capillaries, and the body sends clotting factors to stop the tiny amount of bleeding from the capillaries.

✦ More blood and fluids may come into the area (but this is much less prominent in a back sprain/strain than in an ankle or knee sprain, where you may see a very swollen joint).

✦ Depending on the volume of muscle and ligament tissue that's been sprained/strained, this phase may take only a few days, or may take as long as about two weeks.

PROLIFERATIVE PHASE

The **proliferative phase** begins even while the inflammatory phase is still in progress—often by the third day after an injury. In this phase:

✦ Some of the specialized cells that come to the area of injury, **fibroblasts**, have special properties that enable them to start making a kind of stringy tissue called **collagen**.

✦ As the days pass, with the help of nutrients from the other paramedic cells that came to help, along with oxygen that's brought by the red blood cells, the collagen starts to line up and become oriented.

✦ Other cells and nutrients help make new capillaries and muscle cells.

REMODELING STAGE

In the **remodeling stage**:

✦ The collagen becomes like normal gristle tissue and "glues" the various cells together.

If you were to wait six weeks after a low back sprain/strain and then take a biopsy of the precise area of the back that had sustained the sprain/strain, and if you looked at that biopsy under the microscope, *it would look as if it had never been injured.*

So that's our first important clue to the treatment of a low back sprain/strain: *Even if you did nothing, it would be healed in six weeks.* So why go to the doctor?

If you've ever had a low back sprain/strain, you know that it hurt. A whole lot. You were really stiff and sore. Well, the treatment speeds up the process of healing and shortens the time you feel miserable. So let's get you out of your misery.

PAIN RX: LOW BACK SPRAIN/STRAIN

Home Remedies

Ice. Remember that ice penetrates far deeper than heat, so it gets to the injured area and constricts the capillaries, slowing down the blood flow and reducing the amount of blood cells and fluid leakage from the muscle cells. This won't affect the paramedic cells that will be arriving shortly to begin cleanup and repair. Ice should be used for no more than ten to twenty minutes at a time, and it can be repeated every hour or two for the first day only.

Medication

Analgesics and/or over-the-counter NSAIDs will help relieve pain and inflammation. (Remember, Tylenol does not have anti-inflammatory properties, and aspirin and Excedrin do and should not be taken together with NSAIDs.)

Medical Attention

Get to the doctor ASAP following any injury. This is not a case of "if it looks like a duck (sprain), walks like a duck (sprain), and sounds like a duck (sprain), it must be a duck (sprain)." You need a proper history and physical examination, and you must have x-rays of the lumbar spine. Only Superman has x-ray vision. Doctors don't. X-rays will rule out things that could mimic an acute low back sprain/strain, such as a compression fracture, a facet problem, a developmental bone problem or, heaven forbid, a tumor.

Treatment

Once a doctor verifies that you do have a sprain/strain, you should start physical therapy promptly.

You'll probably start with modalities: a regimen of moist heat (twenty-four hours after an injury, the leaking from capillaries and muscle cells will have stopped), ultrasound, and high-voltage galvanic stimulation (microdyne). These will increase blood flow and allow more paramedic cells, red blood cells, and oxygen to get to the injured area and may help relieve spasm.

Your doctor or physical therapist will show you stretching exercises and gentle flexion and extension exercises (see pages 126 to 133 for examples). As pain and stiffness decrease, you'll add strengthening exercises and aerobic exercises (see pages 123 to 125).

Modalities will be discontinued after one to two weeks (except for moist heat to help tissues get limber before exercising). Massage may be of some benefit, too.

Prognosis

Often, this type of treatment can shorten the healing time for a low back sprain/strain from six weeks to one, two, or three weeks. There is no need to use any type of belt, brace, or fancy orthopaedic garment, and certainly there's no indication for any kind of surgery.

Ligament Injuries

Remember: A tiny amount of motion in the sacroiliac joint can cause severe pain and even mimic the pain of a herniated disc. The pain comes when the cartilage on the sacral side of the joint rubs against the cartilage on the ilium side of the joint. That rubbing occurred because the dense sacroiliac ligaments somehow stretched microscopically.

Pain Rx: Ligament Injuries

Home Remedies

Apply ice directly over the sacroiliac joint for ten to twenty minutes every hour or two for the first day. The ice will help reduce the inflammation in the ligaments.

Medication

Take analgesics and/or OTC NSAIDs.

Medical Attention

I'm going to repeat this for every injury I discuss: It's essential to see a doctor as soon as possible in order to be examined and have x-rays taken.

Treatment

The treatment is designed to do what seems like two paradoxical things: Open the joint and compress the joint. We try to open the joint to prevent the exquisitely painful rubbing, and the home sacroiliac stretching exercises (see pages 131 to 133) are designed to do exactly this. A sacroiliac belt will help compress the joint to try to prevent it from moving while you're up and about. Remember, the sacroiliac joint transmits all the weight of the upper half of the body to the hip and leg, and you want to prevent the shear force discussed in chapter 4.

Some doctors may inject cortisone mixed with lidocaine into the sacroiliac joint because cortisone is a powerful anti-inflammatory medicine. That's a really difficult injection to do successfully. The joint doesn't have a nice wide space the way a knee or shoulder does, so it's very hard to get a needle to "slide" into the joint. What usually happens is that the cortisone and lidocaine often end up infiltrating the surface of the bones (the cortex—the bread of the peanut butter sandwich) and the tissue around it. This may occasionally give some relief.

Physical therapy can be started immediately using modalities including moist heat, ultrasound, and high-voltage galvanic stimulation. Deep transverse friction massage may also help.

Prognosis   Most sprains of the sacroiliac ligament take one to three weeks to resolve with treatment; untreated, they may last six to eight weeks, probably due to the constant irritation from the shear force across the joint.

You, as a patient, have the right to have x-rays ordered or taken as part of your initial examination. Some doctors, at the urging of certain insurance companies, HMOs, et cetera, try to lower the cost of health care by not ordering or doing x-rays initially. That's not good medicine! Certainly, you can play the odds and assume that your pain arose from a simple problem. But that's not smart: I've been surprised too many times by what I've found on back x-rays.

Facet Joint Irritation

Facet joint irritation also occurs because the cartilage on one side of the facet rubs against the cartilage on the other side. Think of it as a miniaturized version of sacroiliac joint irritation. It can occur either because there are arthritic changes within the facet joint or because the facet joint is out of alignment.

PAIN RX: FACET JOINT IRRITATION

Home Remedies
Ice doesn't seem to do much, if any, good for this condition, because the area is small and there's virtually no inflammation.

Medication
Analgesics or anti-inflammatories can be helpful, especially because this problem can be due to arthritic changes.

Medical Attention
See your doctor to be examined and get x-rays.

Treatment
Treatment for facet joint irritation, which is often accompanied by spasm and a sciatic shift, will be similar to that for sacroiliac joint pain.

Physical therapy should begin promptly using moist heat, ultrasound, and sometimes high-voltage galvanic stimulation as well as deep transverse friction massage and regular massage. Stretching and strengthening exercises and even water (pool) exercises should be added when the soreness and stiffness begin to subside.

While a sacroiliac belt may be quite helpful for a sacroiliac strain, there is no type of flexible belt or support that eases facet joint irritation. You can't compress a facet joint the way you can compress a sacroiliac joint, so elasticized wide belts are useless. You might reduce pain with a rigid brace that extends from the armpits to below the pelvis (which would pretty much immobilize the lumbar facet joints), but that's uncomfortable—and expensive—overkill for a condition that's going to get better fairly quickly.

Prognosis

Facet joint irritation, painful though it is, will often clear up in three to six weeks with the vigorous treatment I've outlined. Very occasionally, it doesn't. If it persists, a treatment that may help is the use of facet joint steroid injections given by an anaesthesiologist who specializes in pain management. This technique requires videofluoroscopy to make certain the needle is placed directly in the rather narrow facet joint. When it works, the relief can be quite dramatic.

Herniated Disc

As you learned in chapter 3, a disc can herniate while the posterior longitudinal ligament remains intact, or the disc can burst through the posterior longitudinal ligament and end up lying free in the spinal canal—a free fragment. Both types of herniations will frequently cause identical severe symptoms of radiating leg pain, paresthesias (pins and needles), and numbness. If you have injured your back and have those symptoms, you've most likely run out of luck:

✦ You need to see a doctor *immediately*.

✦ You need x-rays and an MRI scan or CAT scan as soon as possible. If the MRI or CAT scan confirms a herniated disc that correlates precisely with the neurologic examination (which will have revealed a pattern of numbness along a dermatome—the longitudinal band of skin that's supplied by one nerve root; muscle weakness; and possibly diminished reflex), then the game is over: You need surgery.

✦ If these studies are inconclusive, sometimes a myelogram can provide an answer. The symptoms and neurologic examination are usually abnormal enough that there is no need for EMGs and NCTs . . . especially because they may take three weeks to show abnormalities.

I can remember exactly one patient in all my years in orthopaedics who had a documented herniated disc with neurologic changes and confirming x-ray studies, who refused to have surgery, and who recovered. *Every other patient with similar findings who wanted to wait and try physical therapy, injections, and so on, eventually ended up having surgery to remove the offending disc.* Unfortunately, some waited so long that they developed irreversible changes in the muscles and skin supplied by the affected nerve root.

Extruded free fragments of disc may shrivel a bit with the passage of time, and that shriveling—as the water in the fragment evaporates— may result in the free fragment's losing contact with the nerve root or dura. Frankly, you have better chances of winning the lottery than you do of seeing this happen. Believe me, it almost never happens; and waiting and wishing for it to occur only prolongs the time the nerve root remains irritated and reduces your chances for a full and complete recovery of all neurologic function of the nerve root.

Physical therapy is also useless in the treatment of an acute herniated disc. The disc has herniated because a part or all of the nucleus pulposus has broken free. There is no modality, exercise, or massage that's going to make it heal. No injection will help it. No brace or belt will cure it. *Only surgery will correct the problem.*

Once you've decided to have surgery, the gold standard (the surgery with the best success rate and lowest complication rate) is the lumbar laminectomy/microdiscectomy (see page 139). Sometimes it's done as an outpatient procedure where you come in and go home the same day; sometimes it involves a one- to three-day stay afterward. I always recommend going with the gold standard. I can, however, understand why some surgeons are strong advocates of automated percutaneous lumbar microdiscectomy. If they've had lots of experience performing this procedure and there's a pretty good certainty that you don't have a free fragment, you can expect to have a very short recovery.

Hocus Pocus, Nucleus Pulposus

What happens to the space between the vertebral bodies (called the interspace) where the disc resided before it was removed surgically? Believe it or not, sometimes a new nucleus pulposus will form there! I remember one woman patient who literally crawled across the floor into my office because of severe pain she'd developed earlier that day while playing tennis. Her physical examination showed she had a herniated disc; an MRI scan confirmed it. I operated on her two days after her injury and found that the entire nucleus pulposus had burst through the posterior longitudinal ligament and was lying free in the spinal canal, jammed up against the dura and the nerve root. I used special instruments to probe the interspace and found only annulus fibrosus firmly attached to the vertebral end plates (the cartilage on the surface of the bodies). Three years later the same woman came in again with virtually identical symptoms, and a corroborating MRI scan. When I reoperated, I found that the posterior longitudinal ligament was intact but was protruding far into the spinal canal. When I cut into it, once more an entire nucleus pulposus extruded! It's a rare occurrence, but obviously it does happen sometimes.

Usually, after the nucleus pulposus has been removed—and usually the annulus fibrosus is so firmly attached that it can only be removed with

great difficulty—as time passes, the body makes scar tissue in the interspace, and that takes the place of the nucleus. Thus, as time passes, new
lumbar spine x-rays will show that the interspace has become narrower
than it was originally as a result of the loss of the nucleus, which previously literally had pushed the two apposing vertebral bodies apart.

As I mentioned earlier, new techniques are being developed to insert an artificial disc to replace the one that's been removed. If they
work, these artificial discs may help retain flexibility at the operated interspace; they'll definitely prevent the narrowing that occurs with the
passage of time.

Compression Fracture

A fracture—broken bone—is treated by immobilizing the joints on either side of the fractured bone.

> Remember: A compression fracture of a vertebral
> body is wedge shaped, like a piece of pie, as a result
> of crushing of the anterior (front) part of the vertebral
> body by very strong flexion (bending) forces.

You need to see a doctor right away. The physical examination, as you
learned in chapter 3, will often show intense, localized, unremitting pain
even at rest. Of course, x-rays will quickly confirm the diagnosis. (You saw
diagnostic studies of compression fractures in chapter 3, figures 3–15,
3–16, and 3–17.)

Not only is physical therapy of no value in the treatment, but here it
can actually cause harm. You don't want moist heat because you don't
want to increase the bleeding at the fracture site. You don't want the
other modalities for the same reason. You certainly don't want massage,
because you don't want the fracture to shift.

The proper treatment is a back brace. The brace will be designed to keep you in a posture that involves being straight or even with a little extra lordosis (the C-shaped curve seen from the side where the mid-part of the C faces toward the abdomen). This posture helps keep the compressed vertebral body from compressing even more. Sometimes, though not always, it may even help to pull apart the compressed vertebral body and help to restore the height of the anterior (front) part. A number of types of back braces are used for this. One type is a lightweight aluminum modular one called a Jewett brace. A second type is a custom-molded lightweight plastic one that's like a clamshell. Some people even still use a Knight spinal brace made of steel straps covered with leather, or its larger version, the Knight-Taylor brace, for compression fractures in the thoracic and high upper lumbar spine.

After the compression fracture has been diagnosed and the measurements made for the brace, you need to do several things until the brace is fabricated:

✦ Lie *flat*, only rolling like a log onto your sides.

✦ You don't want to twist (that's why you roll like a log). It could make the two halves of the fracture shear or shift.

✦ You certainly don't want to sit: That will increase flexion forces and possibly create more compression.

✦ You'll also want to eat lightly for a day or two. The blood that leaks will mostly go anteriorly, toward the front, and it will pool just behind the lining of the abdominal cavity. That irritates the lining, which makes a reflex irritation of the bowels—and they get quiet and sometimes don't work. The same occasionally holds true for the bladder.

It should take only one to three days for the brace to be fabricated. Occasionally, patients get admitted to the hospital until then. Often, however, the patient is allowed to go home (lying down on the backseat of the car), stay flat in bed, log-roll onto the side when eating, and only get out of bed for quick trips to the bathroom.

Finger fractures take three weeks to heal. Wrist fractures take six weeks to heal. Compression fractures of the lumbar spine take twelve weeks to heal, and *there is nothing you can do to speed that up*. So you'll wear the brace for twelve weeks. You'll put it on and take it off while you're lying down, but once it's on, you may be up and about as much as you want. You can even sit with the brace on. But you may not drive: You'd have to turn to the right and left to look over your shoulder, and the brace is poor at preventing shearing. After twelve weeks, you'll be weaned from the brace over a period of one to two weeks, because the paraspinal muscles will have gotten weak from not having to work while the brace took over to keep you erect.

Once you're weaned from the brace, you may, as I always told my patients, do anything that's legal or moral.

Painful Coccyx

You've learned that the coccyx can be contused (bruised) or fractured. Both injures are treated the same way. A painful coccyx is exquisitely tender when any pressure is applied to it, and sitting is the only thing that applies pressure to the coccyx. So the first thing to do to relieve pain is very simple: Take the pressure off the coccyx when you sit. Doctors used to have patients sit on rubber doughnuts, with the center of the doughnuts supposedly keeping the coccyx suspended. But the pressure of the doughnut on the surrounding area often creates pain at the coccyx anyway. Now a rolled towel is used instead.

PAIN RX: PAINFUL COCCYX

Home Remedies	Use a rolled towel whenever you sit.
Medication	Analgesics and OTC NSAIDs.

Medical Attention	X-rays are needed to determine if the coccyx is fractured; occasionally the fracture may be displaced so one coccygeal bone is shifted.
Treatment	Physical therapy should begin promptly. Whirlpool often helps relieve discomfort when the coccyx is either contused or fractured, and it can be started immediately. Ultrasound can be added for a contused coccyx but not for a fractured coccyx. If pain persists for months in the case of a fractured coccyx, on very rare occasions an injection of cortisone and lidocaine can be given directly at the area of soreness, but this must be done with great care, and it should only rarely be repeated. In the past, sometimes surgery was performed to remove the coccyx; this is almost never done today.
Prognosis	Usually, the pain will resolve within four to six weeks.

Junior Doctor's Merit Badge Checkpoint

MAKING A ROLLED TOWEL

How do you take away pressure from the coccyx when sitting?

Take a bath towel, fold it in half lengthwise and then roll it up into a log. (We simply call it a "rolled towel".) Sit on a firm, hard chair. Place the rolled towel just behind and under your knees on your chair. **(Fig.6–1)** You've just turned the rolled towel into the fulcrum of a seesaw, and the buttocks will be elevated the tiny amount needed to take pressure off the coccyx.

Figure 6-1

Rolled Towel for Painful Coccyx

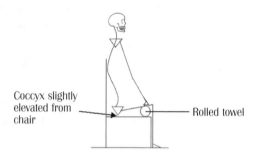

Coccyx slightly elevated from chair ————→   ———— Rolled towel

Degenerative Disc Disease and Degenerative Arthritis

Although degenerative disc disease theoretically involves just the intervertebral discs and degenerative arthritis theoretically involves the facet joints, in real life they are, as the song says, kind of like love and marriage: You rarely have one without the other. As a disc degenerates, losing its water of hydration, it starts to collapse because it can't hold up the weight of the entire body above it. When this happens, the interspace in which the disc resides becomes narrower. (**Fig. 6–2**) As the interspace narrowing happens at the anterior (front) half of the vertebra at the body, narrowing starts to occur posteriorly at the back half of the vertebra, at the facet joint. But because of the shape and inclination of the facet joint on each side of the vertebra at that level, the superior facet (of the vertebra above) starts to slide down a tiny bit on the inferior facet of the vertebra below. We say the joint is no longer **congruent**, and so the two parts rub against each other, wearing away the lining cartilage and causing **hypertrophy** (the formation of extra bone).

Figure 6-2

X-rays Showing Degenerative Arthritis and Degenerative Disc Disease

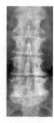 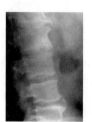

Front view   Side view

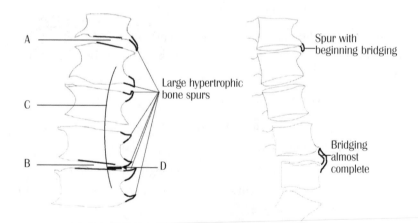

A — Large hypertrophic bone spurs

C

B — D

Spur with beginning bridging

Bridging almost complete

X-ray Vision

On the front view, notice the asymmetric disc degeneration at **(A)** and **(B)** which has resulted in a degenerative scoliosis **(C)**. There is also a vacuum disc phenomenon, replacement of the water of the disc by nitrogen gas, at **(D)**.

On the side view, notice how the anterior longitudinal ligament has turned to bone at two different areas, creating bone spurs. Both areas have a) - shaped appearance because the annulus fibrosus of the disc bulged circumferentially, and when it protruded anteriorly (toward the abdomen), it forced the anterior longitudinal ligament to bulge anteriorly as well.

Two things can happen from a combination of degenerative disc disease and degenerative arthritis:

1. You can experience a sudden onset of pain after an activity such as lifting, carrying, or the like.

2. You can have chronic (for more than six months) nagging back pain accompanied by stiffness and possibly leg pain.

There are some differences in their treatment, but, again, treatment for both begins with a physical examination by the doctor and lumbar spine x-rays.

If your pain came on suddenly:

✦ You need to be carefully evaluated to make certain that you don't have nerve root irritation.

✦ An MRI scan or CAT scan can quickly show whether or not there is impingement of a nerve root. Occasionally a myelogram may be needed.

✦ If there is no evidence of nerve root irritation, then the symptoms can be attacked vigorously with prescription-strength NSAIDs and physical therapy.

✦ All modalities (see pages 118 to 122) except ice can be used initially.

✦ Sometimes McKenzie extension exercises (see page 124) can give relief over a period of time.

+ Massage may feel nice but often isn't of much help.

+ Dynamic stabilization exercises may also help, and, of course, home exercises (see pages 126 to 133) are essential.

+ As symptoms subside, aerobic exercises including water (pool) therapy are often beneficial. The goal is to restore and increase flexibility, which in turn relieves pain and stiffness.

Degenerative arthritis and **degenerative disc disease** slowly progress over the years. Sometimes this progression slows down or even stops; less often it rapidly becomes worse. The forms of nonoperative, or conservative, treatment that I've been describing should relieve the *symptoms*, such as pain and stiffness, which this progression causes. Unfortunately, nothing you can do at home will reverse these conditions and make the bone spurs get smaller or a disc space get wider. Only surgery can attempt to affect the continued progression of bony changes.

If you've had chronic lower back pain and stiffness for more than six months, you need somewhat different treatment:

+ Your pain may radiate into one or both legs, but you shouldn't have neurologic symptoms of numbness or paresthesias (pins and needles). An MRI or CAT scan may be ordered to help rule out nerve root impingement.

+ A bone scan may be done to see if there is an area of active arthritis. Electromyograms and nerve conduction tests may also help rule out nerve root irritation.

+ Treatment will need to be more gentle, because chronic long-term pain means that most likely you have suffered considerable loss of mobility—in other words, stiffness—due to prolonged arthritic irritation.

✦ Moist heat should be used both in physical therapy and at home. In fact, using moist heat at home for twenty minutes three or four times daily just by itself can help loosen tight muscles.

✦ The other modalities will have limited benefit since there is no classic inflammation as is seen in an acute injury. Water (pool) therapy can be started early and many times helps overcome stiffness. Dynamic stabilization exercises and flexion exercises (see pages 128 to 130) often help, although some patients may get better relief with McKenzie extension exercises (see page 124).

✦ Prescription NSAIDs may help relieve both pain and stiffness.

✦ As improvement occurs, aerobic exercises including walking will be very beneficial.

✦ Orthopaedic belts, braces, and the like will not be of any value: There's nothing to compress, and immobilization will only promote stiffness, not relieve it.

Spinal Stenosis

Spinal stenosis, as you learned in chapter 4, is the extreme form of degenerative arthritis and degenerative disc disease.

Remember: The thickened undersurface of the lamina, the thickened ligamentum flavum, the hypertrophic bony spurring of the pedicles (pillars) and facets, and the posterior bulging of the discs can all combine to impinge upon, indent, and kink the dura—which covers the central group of spinal nerve roots in the spinal canal—and/or the exiting spinal nerve root as it goes through the intervertebral foramen (the space between adjacent pedicles).

✦ We diagnose spinal stenosis beginning with a careful history, which may reveal an increase in symptoms when the patient extends (bends backward) or walks—spinal claudication.

✦ Physical examination often demonstrates neurologic changes including diminished or absent sensation, muscle weakness, reflex changes, and so forth.

✦ Lumbar spine x-rays show advanced degenerative arthritis and degenerative disc disease.

✦ An MRI or CAT scan will show the thickened laminae, ligamentum flavum, facet hypertrophy, disc bulging, and the resultant impingement, indentation, and/or kinking of the dura and nerve roots.

✦ A myelogram will likewise show the indentation of the dura and nerve root impingement. In fact, the myelogram can be very dramatic, showing the dura looking like an hourglass because it has been so constricted.

✦ Electromyograms and nerve conduction tests will confirm nerve root irritation.

You also learned that spinal stenosis can cause unremitting back pain, radiating leg pain that may be constant or intermittent, paresthesias (pins and needles), numbness, and muscle weakness. Sometimes nonoperative treatment may relieve symptoms; other times it doesn't, however, and then surgery is necessary. The nonoperative treatment for spinal stenosis involves the same things that were just described for the treatment of *chronic* degenerative arthritis and degenerative disc disease, with one important difference: McKenzie exercises and home prone and standing extension exercises must *not* be used, because they will result in increased impingement on the dura and nerve roots.

If nonoperative treatment does not result in any improvement after a period of three or four months, then surgery is the proper next step. The operation for spinal stenosis is much more extensive than a lumbar microdiscectomy or a lumbar laminectomy. Because spinal stenosis invariably extends over several vertebrae, the surgery for it must also involve work on several vertebrae. The thickened ligamentum flavum must be removed, the thickened part of the laminae must be removed, and the bony spurring of the facets and pedicles must be ground down using miniature high-speed burrs.

Sometimes the hourglass constriction of the dura is so extensive that the surgeon must remove the spinous process (the chimney) and the entire middle part of the right and left laminae (roofs) where they meet in the center, along with all of the ligamentum flavum above and below the vertebra. (**Fig. 6–3**) Unfortunately, doing this trades one set of problems for another; still, the benefits from doing this extensive "unroofing" usually outweigh the side effects. Here's the problem:

Figure 6-3

X-ray Showing Complete Laminectomy for Spinal Stenosis

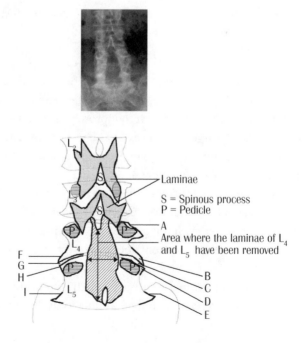

Laminae

S = Spinous process
P = Pedicle

A
Area where the laminae of L₄ and L₅ have been removed

F
G
H
I

B
C
D
E

X-ray Vision

The spurs at the corners **(B)** and **(F)** of the fourth lumbar vertebra, and the spurs at the corners **(D)** and **(H)** of the fifth lumbar vertebra on the x-ray on page 168 occurred as a reaction to the markedly advanced degeneration of the disc between those two vertebrae **(C)**, **(G)**. In fact, it was that advanced degenerative disc disease with the accompanying spurs which necessitated the complete removal of the laminae of the fourth and fifth lumbar vertebrae. Note the additional spurs at **(A)**, **(E)**, and **(I)**.

You may have noticed that the pedicles (the walls of our vertebral house) and the laminae form a rigid arch extending up, across, and back down to the vertebral body. This arch is really strong and provides a solid, rigid support for the paraspinal muscles, allowing them to contract and pull the spine up straight. There is not even the tiniest motion or yielding of the laminae no matter how much weight you bend over to pick up or how forcefully you straighten up.

If the spinous process and entire middle part of the laminae are removed, there's no longer an arch. (**Fig. 6–4**)

Figure 6-4

"Blueprint" Drawing of Complete Laminectomy

Spinous process and laminae removed

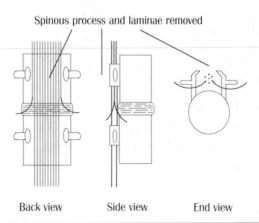

Back view   Side view   End view

Although that removes the cause of the hourglass constriction, it also takes away the solid, rigid support for the paraspinal muscles. That may result in persistent backache as the muscles function during all the activities of daily living. The improvement in neurologic function is almost always worth this trade-off. The backache may need to be treated by the use of a custom-made back brace, which will help support the low back and ease the work of the paraspinal muscles.

Stress Fracture

You won't know you have a stress fracture; you'll just know that you have some back pain that's come on gradually and intermittently and is getting worse. You see the doctor, who examines you and finds one really tender spot centered over one vertebra. Lumbar spine x-rays may often not show anything; sometimes they may show some increased sclerosis (extra bone) in a pedicle. A three-phase bone scan will quickly give the diagnosis: There will be increased uptake of the radioactive dye in one small area, usually of a pedicle. An MRI scan will also show a stress fracture, but it costs three times as much as a bone scan.

To treat a stress fracture:

✦ You'll be fitted with a custom-made back brace, often the light-weight, aluminum, modular Jewett brace, for a period of twelve weeks. Just as with a compression fracture, the brace should be put on and taken off while you lie down; with the brace on, you can do all activities—including driving in most cases.

✦ Analgesics such as aspirin or Tylenol or OTC NSAIDs such as Advil will help.

✦ Physical therapy is contraindicated, meaning do not do it at all.

✦ After the stress fracture has healed—and sometimes a second bone scan is needed to confirm this—it takes one to two weeks to be weaned from the brace and resume full activities without restriction. Remember: This is an injury that's often seen in athletes, so it's important to have it heal fully before resuming sports and athletic activities.

Spondylolysis and Spondylolisthesis

You don't awaken one morning with back pain and say, "Golly, I must have spondylolysis or spondylolisthesis." In fact, you may be well into middle age and never know you have it . . . until you have your first set of lumbar spine x-rays.

 Remember: Spondylolysis is the absence of bone in the special area of the pedicle (the pillar) called the pars interarticularis, the broken neck of the Scottie dog. It's rarely just on one side; usually it's bilateral. And you must have bilateral spondylolysis before you can start to have spondylolisthesis, the slipping forward of the body of the vertebra above in relation to the vertebra below.

Spondylolisthesis itself doesn't hurt. Spondylolysis does. Remember how I mentioned the fact that the pedicles and laminae make a nice rigid arch? Well, if there's nothing connecting the laminae and upper half of the pedicles to the lower half of the pedicles and vertebral body, that floating upper arch serves as a lousy anchor for the paraspinal muscles when they contract while you're bending, lifting, or carrying. That floating lamina works about as well as if you were wearing roller skates on a slippery surface, and you were alone on one side of a rope, playing tug-of-war against a dozen 250-pound weight lifters.

You've also learned that, because of some laws of physics, as the upper vertebral body slips forward, the disc between it and the vertebral body below gets pushed back circumferentially, protruding into the spinal canal, and may impinge against the dura and/or nerve roots and cause nerve root irritation.

So you develop back pain for some reason, you go to the doctor, you're examined, the doctor may find signs of hamstring tightness (the muscles on the back of the thigh), and lumbar spine x-rays are taken. Voilà! The Scottie Dogs are seen to have broken necks at one vertebra; usually some slipping of the vertebral body is also present, and they may actually be slipping 25 to 50 percent (Grade I to Grade III).

If you've never had back pain before—and be honest!—then even with a Grade II spondylolisthesis, you may be able to be treated for a back sprain/strain . . . as long as you don't also have any abnormalities on neurologic examination. Physical therapy modalities (see pages 118 to 122) may be used; McKenzie extension exercises (see page 124) will be very helpful. Avoid massage and all flexion exercises, because flexion, or bending forward, is what makes spondylolisthesis slip and causes symptoms. In addition to routine lumbar spine x-rays, you'll need to have flexion and extension lateral x-rays. These are x-rays of the lumbar spine taken from the side while you bend forward (flex), stand straight, and bend backward (extend). If they show that the spondylolisthesis increases as you bend forward, and gets less (we say reduces) when you extend, then it's unstable and it's guaranteed to continue progressing. And *that* means that even if you've never had back pain before and this is your first episode, physical therapy is out: You need surgery. Surgery is necessary for symptomatic spondylolisthesis regardless of whether or not it's unstable. If it's stable, but persists in being symptomatic despite a several-month period of good nonoperative treatment, something isn't right. Tissues are slowly yielding, and it will become unstable. The surgery that's done for spondylolisthesis is a spine fusion. A variety of techniques are used, but they all have one goal: to prevent further slipping. Sometimes, some of the slipping can be reduced during surgery, but that's a secondary consideration.

To fuse spondylolisthesis, we must bridge from the vertebra above the vertebra with the broken Scottie dog neck to the vertebra below it. (**Fig. 6–5**) The physics involved is simple:

✦ We connect two stable vertebrae, each with normal partes interarticulares, one above and one below the one that's slipping, so that the solid body-pedicle-lamina unit above the slip is connected to a similarly solid body-pedicle-lamina unit below, and further slipping is impossible.

Figure 6-5

"Blueprint" Drawing of Fusion for Spondylolisthesis

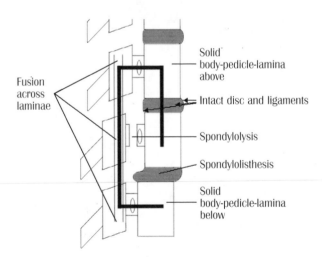

✦ The solid unit above is connected to the slipped body of the **listhetic** vertebra (the vertebra containing the Scottie dog with the "broken neck") by the anterior and posterior longitudinal ligaments and the intact annulus fibrosus (and nucleus pulposus) of the disc between them. But since the slip occurs at the *lower* end of the vertebral body, there's no slipping at the upper part, and that's why this new solid unit can't slip any further. Instrumentation is almost always used for extra rigidity. (**Fig. 6–6**)

Figure 6-6

Side View X-Ray Showing Fusion for Spondylolisthesis

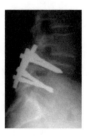

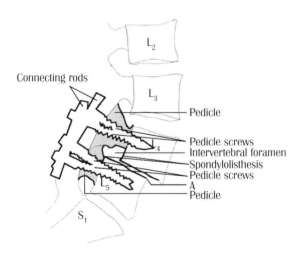

X-ray Vision

The fourth lumbar vertebra in the x-ray on page 174 has slipped forward more than 25% in relation to the fifth, therefore this is a Grade II spondylolisthesis. In this patient, the anterior superior (front upper) edge of the body of the fifth lumbar vertebra (**A**) did not round off.

The surgeon who performed this fusion used a technique different from that which I described: Only the two vertebrae involved in the spondylolisthesis were fused.

✦ Recovery may be slow—anywhere from three months to a year. A custom-made back brace is necessary during recovery to prevent abnormal stresses on the healing area.

✦ Physical therapy can be started after recovery is complete. It should include strengthening, conditioning, and aerobic exercises to build up strength and flexibility.

If there is symptomatic spondylolysis and no spondylolisthesis, surgery is also the proper treatment. A spine fusion is performed and may involve, among other things, scraping out the broken necks of the Scottie dogs and packing them with marrow bone as well as inserting pedicle screws. Recovery and postrecovery treatment is the same as described above.

Degenerative Spondylolisthesis

Remember: Degenerative spondylolisthesis occurs because of severe degeneration of a pair of facet joints at one vertebra, causing the upper half of the facet to slide down the the lower half. The pedicles and the partes interarticulares are intact. (The Scottie dog's neck is normal.) This degenerative

> facet slipping can cause narrowing of the
> intervertebral foramina (the openings through
> which the spinal nerve roots exit from the spinal
> canal) and forward slipping of the vertebra in
> relation to the one below, with backward rolling of
> the disc—just as in classic spondylolisthesis.

When degenerative spondylolisthesis becomes symptomatic, it usually comes on gradually.

✦ The physical examination may show neurologic changes. The lumbar spine x-rays will show the problem, including the facet abnormalities, the foraminal narrowing, and the spondylolisthesis. An MRI or CAT scan will show any evidence of nerve root impingement. Electromyograms and nerve conduction tests will confirm nerve root irritation, if it has occurred.

✦ If there's no nerve root irritation, prescription NSAIDs and a trial of physical therapy are indicated. Modalities including moist heat (see page 118), and ultrasound (see page 120), McKenzie extension exercises (see page 124), water (pool) therapy (see page 125), and possibly a back brace may help to alleviate symptoms.

✦ If there is nerve root irritation, or if a trial of physical therapy doesn't help, then surgery is the correct treatment. The facet joints will need to be smoothed, bone spurs will need to be removed, the foramina will need to be widened using high-speed miniature burrs, and a spine fusion may need to be done with instrumentation.

✦ After surgery, a custom-made back brace will be necessary, and recovery may take from three months to a year. After recovering, the patient will need strengthening and aerobic (conditioning) exercises (see pages 123–125).

Transitional Vertebrae

If you've hurt your back or developed lumbosacral back pain for some reason, and you've gone to the doctor and been examined and had lumbar spine x-rays taken, and if those x-rays showed that the first sacral vertebra (S_1 in medical shorthand) really looked like a lumbar vertebra and had little, discrete lumbar-looking transverse processes, you have **lumbarization of S_1**. Now the sacrum, the base of the spine, acts as an anchor for the paraspinal muscles, just as the giant concrete structures at the ends of the Golden Gate Bridge anchor the suspension cables that hold up the bridge. If S_1 is lumbarized, it can't perform its assigned function as well as it should, and that can cause back pain.

The physical examination will often show that the tenderness is located over the first sacral vertebra, while neurologic examination will be normal. The diagnosis will leap out from the front view x-ray of the lumbar spine, and usually no other tests or studies are needed.

Treatment for lumbarization of S_1 is nonoperative. You've essentially suffered a back sprain/strain, and the treatment is that described for sprains and strains at the beginning of this chapter.

On the other hand, if we change our scenario so that the x-rays showed a markedly enlarged transverse process on one or both sides of the fifth lumbar vertebra (L_5), we have an entirely different ball game. **Hemisacralization** (one enlarged transverse process) or **complete sacralization** (both transverse processes) of L_5 can cause exquisite back pain as well as pain radiating down one or both legs because of actual mechanical rubbing of the enlarged transverse process against the transverse process of S_1, the adjacent part of the ilium bone, or both.

A trial of physical therapy may work, and the pain may resolve. With pain of acute onset, all modalities may help; deep transverse friction massage as well as massage may help break up spasm. Stretching and strengthening exercises can reduce stiffness and pain. Home exercises also help and can be done three or four times daily. NSAIDs, either over the counter or prescription strength, can help reduce the inflammation that results from the mechanical rubbing and thus relieve pain.

Rarely, videofluoroscopically guided cortisone injections may be needed. Also rarely, a custom-made back brace that comes down low onto the hips may be needed.

In the rare cases where back pain and possibly leg pain persist despite vigorous nonoperative treatment, then a spine fusion may become necessary, especially if the transverse process is clearly rubbing against the sacrum, ilium, or both. Only the fifth lumbar and first sacral vertebrae need to be fused, with special attention taken to fuse the transverse process. Alternatively, some advocate shortening the enlarged transverse process, which eliminates the mechanical rubbing and avoids having to do a fusion. The recovery from that latter procedure is relatively quick: often six to ten weeks. The recovery following a fusion is three to six months.

Chapter Seven

HOW WE DON'T TREAT THE BACK
WHAT DOESN'T WORK—AND WHY

I've just spent several chapters telling you what works in the treatment of lower back pain. All these treatments have been scientifically studied and tested, and they're based on rational, scientific, medical thinking. Now I'm going to tell you about some things that really don't work. I realize that some of you may have used some of these things over the years when you had back pain. You may even have experienced relief of your pain shortly after using them. You may be unhappy to see a favorite remedy listed here and think that I've taken leave of my senses.

I'd like you to be patient and read carefully what I'm about to tell you. I think you'll find that if you reflect on a favorite remedy that has no scientific justification and truly can't do what it purports to, you may realize how helpful to the process of healing is the mighty power of suggestion. If your injury wasn't very severe and you desperately wanted to get better as fast as possible, and you used one of these remedies, your faith in it may have made it seem to work for you. You'll see as you read on, that many, many patients improve when their treatment has been nothing more than a sugar pill or a pretend medical device.

After you've read this chapter, if you still want to continue to use a favorite remedy I've described here, go ahead and do so—as long as it's not bankrupting you, prolonging your pain, or leading to more severe problems.

Bed Rest

Did you notice in chapters 5 and 6 that I never mentioned bed rest? If so, did you think that I'd become sloppy or forgetful? Well, if you did, you're wrong! Why didn't I tell you to use bed rest if you had an acute low back sprain/strain, degenerative disc disease, or degenerative arthritis? Everyone knows that sometimes those conditions *really* hurt a whole lot, and it feels so good to lie down and stay in bed for a few days . . . because it hurts so much to move, to get out of bed, and to walk around.

Well, to be honest with you, orthopaedic surgeons were a bit slow in learning to recognize that bed rest is bad. It was used often when I was doing my residency and even in the early years of my private practice. But eventually, even orthopaedic surgeons woke up and learned what much of the medical community had realized years earlier.

Back in the 1930s, if you had an appendectomy, a hernia repair, or your gallbladder removed, you stayed in the hospital a long time. And you stayed on bed rest, often for two to three weeks. Then World War II came, and soldiers were being injured in the European and Asian theaters of war, but they were needed in battle. Bright combat surgeons noticed that if they got their patients out of bed rapidly, the soldiers recovered faster and had fewer complications. But *rapidly* still meant staying in bed for several days, and that lasted well into the 1980s. Now patients having those same operations are out of bed the moment they get out of the recovery room.

We now know that staying in bed twenty hours a day when you have back pain does no more good for your back than does lying down for a few hours and then getting up and moving about. In one study, patients with acute back pain who were on bed rest twenty hours a day were no more improved two weeks and twelve weeks later than were patients with acute lower back pain who had been allowed to be active. Much more importantly, bed rest results in the rapid loss of muscle tone, and in the loss of muscle mass after two weeks. It may lead to circulatory problems such as the development of blood clots in the veins in the calf, which is called **deep vein thrombosis** or **thrombophlebitis**.

So if you've developed acute lower back pain, it's severe, and it hurts to do anything, don't take to your bed! That doesn't mean that you can't lie down for an hour or two once or twice a day for the first day or two. Lying down on your back does help unload the spine. (This means it doesn't have much to support or hold up, like the entire upper half of your body.) But don't just lie flat on your back. Bend your knees and hips, place a pillow under your calves and a long pillow under your head and upper back. You're now in the reclining chair position, also known by its fancy medical name, **semi-Fowler's**. (**Fig. 7–1**) You can also lie on your side, curled up in a semi-fetal position, with a pillow between your knees. (**Fig. 7–2**)

Figure 7-1

Semi-Fowler's Position

Legs parallel to bed

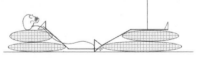

Figure 7-2

Side-Lying Bed Rest

Pillow

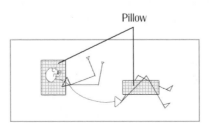

Transcutaneous Electric Nerve Stimulation

Transcutaneous electric nerve stimulation, known by many as **TENS**, is a treatment that many doctors prescribe but that, unfortunately, doesn't really do anything. It's based on the gate theory of pain control. As you know, nerves go from the spinal cord to every part of the body. There are two types of these nerves: **motor nerves**, which supply the muscles and make them contract, and **sensory nerves**, which supply the skin and deeper structures with feeling. Sensory nerves have many different types of endings, so they can sense pain, pressure, heat, cold, stretch, and so forth.

If a pain sensory nerve ending senses pain, it sends an electrical signal back up its nerve. This nerve goes to the spinal cord, so the electric signal then travels up the spinal cord to the brain, which registers that a particular part of the body hurts. In the spine, muscles, ligaments, facets, discs, and vertebrae all have nerve endings that sense pain. When the back is injured, the pain endings of the nerves supplying the painful structures send electrical signals up these nerves to the spinal cord. The gate theory says that there are nerve gates in the spinal cord. It's possible for the brain to send signals down the spinal cord to these nerve gates and tell them to close, thus blocking the pain signals. It's also possible for the brain to send signals down the spinal cord to tell those nerve gates to open—allowing the pain signals to zoom up to the brain. If you can find a way to block these nerve impulses by making the gate close, the gate theory says you can block the perception of pain.

A transcutaneous electric nerve stimulator, or TENS unit, is a battery-powered device that supposedly sends electrical signals **transcutaneously** (through the skin) and down through the other layers of fatty tissue and muscle to the spinal nerve gate. These electrical signals theoretically close the gate and thus block the pain impulses that are arising from the injured, painful parts of the back and that are trying to go up the spinal cord to the brain.

The actual TENS unit is about the size of a package of cigarettes. It contains electronic circuits that generate a special electric pattern, or wave, that's been specifically engineered to travel through the skin, the subcutaneous tissue, the lumbodorsal fascia, the paraspinal muscles, the ligamentum flavum and laminae, and the dura, then to penetrate the spinal cord and create the electrical signal required to close the gate. Electric leads, or wires, go from the TENS unit to small self-sticking pads, which are similar to those used when you have an electrocardiogram and are attached to the skin at specific sites on the spine. A control on the TENS unit allows the wearer to turn it on and off and to set the intensity of the electrical signal that's being sent through the skin. The wearer sets the intensity level by trial and error, trying to find the proper intensity that blocks the pain impulses. That's the theory.

But that's not reality. In medicine, we evaluate whether a new form of treatment will work by doing a scientific study in which there is only one variable: the thing being studied.

Junior Doctor's Merit Badge Checkpoint

In a **double-blind study**, patients being treated for an illness or condition don't know whether their treatment is actual medication or whether it's a pretend treatment or **placebo**: a sugar pill that looks just like the one being tested. In other words, the patient is blind regarding the treatment because he or she doesn't know whether the test treatment or the placebo treatment is being given. In addition, patients are assigned to receive either the real medicine being tested or the placebo.

After the course of treatment is completed, doctors evaluate all the patients who have been treated by the test medicine and by the placebo. Like the patients, the doctors have no idea which patients received the pill. They, too, are blind, which makes the study a **randomized**

> **double-blind study.** This is the most rigorous and scientific kind of test: The evaluation of the treatment is completely unbiased since *neither patient nor evaluator has any idea which treatment—test medicine or placebo—was received.* Only after the code, which identifies what each individual patient received, is broken is it finally possible to determine whether the medicine being tested really worked or whether the placebo worked just as well.

A group of researchers in Ontario, Canada, studied a series of 324 patients who had acute episodes of lower back pain. Half the patients randomly were fitted with TENS units of the type I described above. The other half were randomly selected and received fake TENS units. These fake TENS units were made to look and weigh exactly the same as the real ones. They even needed to have batteries inserted daily because they were constructed to wear down the batteries at the same rate as the real TENS units. The fake units did not deliver any kind of electric impulses; the real ones did, just as I've described above.

After the study was completed and the patients were all evaluated in this randomized double-blind study, the code was broken. Guess what? There was no statistical difference between the patients who wore the *fake* TENS units and the patients with the *real* TENS units! If fake, or placebo, treatment produces results equal to that of real treatment, *then the treatment being studied is of no real value.* It just goes to show how great the power of suggestion is.

Trigger Point Injections

Trigger points are individual tiny spots of sharp, intense pain that are said to occur in muscles or gristle tissue. These tiny spots are supposed to be markedly irritable and are diagnosed when the doctor palpates (touches or pushes) the area and the patient jumps and says *ouch!* That's what is called a **subjective response** in medicine. A subjective response or subjective finding is something that the patient controls completely. The best example is the child who complains of severe pain that clears up instantly the moment it's kissed and made better.

An **objective finding**, on the other hand, is something over which the patient has no control. One of the best examples is an x-ray: A patient may complain bitterly of pain in a particular bone after a fall and may be convinced that it's broken. But the x-ray may be negative, showing no signs of a fracture, regardless of how vocally the patient complains.

Those who believe in trigger points feel that these trigger points are related to muscle bands that become very tight or taut and can last for months if untreated. They also feel that trigger points will be masked in the initial stages of an acute back sprain/strain because of diffuse inflammation and muscle pain. They treat trigger points by injecting them with cortisone and a local anesthetic, such as lidocaine. Many times, a single injection doesn't cure the problem, and so the injection is repeated after a varying period of time.

There are a number of problems with the concept of trigger points. First, as I've noted, they are purely subjective. I've seen patients who claimed to have trigger points. As I palpated their backs, they'd jump or flinch when I supposedly found the exact triggers. Sometimes I'd mark those trigger points with a felt-tipped pen so I'd know the exact spot. If I then performed other parts of the physical examination, allowing several minutes to go by, and then returned to palpating the back, I *always* noted a fascinating finding. I would not say anything as I palpated, so the patient had no clue when I reached the previously marked spots. Without exception, the patient *always* failed to say "ouch!" or flinch or twitch when I palpated over the marked spots but did say "ouch!" or flinch or twitch as I palpated over different, unmarked spots. No one has ever claimed that trigger points jump around every several minutes, which is what I'd have had to believe if I had believed the patients' subjective complaints.

Second, biopsies have been taken of purported trigger points and have been carefully studied. No abnormality of the tissue has ever been found. No abnormal substances have been identified in the biopsied material. In addition, biopsies of the tissue of trigger points are indistinguishable from biopsies of normal tissue.

Third, if the same trigger point is repeatedly injected with cortisone and lidocaine, the cumulative effect of multiple cortisone injections in the same spot is that there is shriveling up and scarring of the muscle tissue. That scar tissue has none of the resilience or elasticity of normal muscle tissue, and so one problem is traded for a second, more severe problem.

Fourth, randomized double-blind studies have shown that trigger point injections don't work. One such study was performed by orthopaedic surgeons at George Washington University Medical Center in Washington, DC. In this study, patients who were diagnosed by their physicians as having trigger points were sent to the researchers for treatment. The physicians who referred the patients had no idea that a randomized double-blind study was being performed. The patients were randomly assigned to one of four groups, each of which received "trigger point injections." The patients had no idea what they actually received, because the injections were given to trigger points on the back and, unlike your mother when you were a child, the patients didn't have eyes on the backs of their heads.

The four random groups received the following:

+ **Group 1** received a classic trigger point injection of cortisone and lidocaine.

+ **Group 2** received an injection of only lidocaine.

+ For **Group 3**, a needle was inserted and nothing was injected.

+ And then there was **Group 4**. Their injection consisted of spraying the area with a cold spray then pressing the plastic cap covering the needle against the skin. No needle was inserted, nothing was injected, but everything else was done as if the patient were receiving an injection.

The results were fascinating: While about 40 percent of the patients who received the classic trigger point injections of cortisone and lidocaine said that they experienced complete relief, a whopping *66 percent of patients who merely had the plastic needle cap pressed against their skin said they had complete relief of their symptoms.* In fact, the combined positive response of those patients receiving either the injection of cortisone and lidocaine or the injection of only lidocaine was 42 percent, while the combined positive response was 63 percent for those getting either a needle stick or the plastic needle cover pressed against the skin. Once more, the placebo, the fake treatment, had far better results than the "real" treatment.

Now, it's important to distinguish between these trigger point injections of cortisone and lidocaine and the injections I described in chapters 5 and 6 that are given into facet joints or sacroiliac joints. The latter injections are given into objectively diagnosed areas that have real pathology.

Magnets

In chapter 2, you learned how scanner works. You saw that it contains a huge permanent magnet that generates an intense magnetic field, and that this magnetic field is so strong it causes all of the electrical charges of the atoms of water molecules to line up in the same plane or direction. You learned that a second very powerful electromagnet is then rapidly turned on and off, and that each time it's turned on, the electrical charges jump to a new energy state, while each time it's turned off, they return to their original energy state.

You also learned that a good MRI scanner has a permanent magnet that generates a magnetic field sixty thousand times the level of the background magnetic field of the earth. We call this, in electromagnetic shorthand, a magnet strength of 1.5 Tesla.

Quick History Lesson

For you history buffs, Nikola Tesla was a Serbian American inventor, scientist, and electrical engineer who had more than seven hundred patents and who developed, among many other things, the rotating magnetic field principle. The original MRI scanners had a magnetic field of 0.5 Tesla, twenty thousand times the earth's background magnetic field. They worked—and are still in use, with considerably updated computer software. They make fairly decent pictures, but because they're relatively weak magnets, they lack some of the fine resolution of the bigger machines. Currently, new scanners are being developed with magnets powerful enough to generate fields of 2.0 and even 2.5 Tesla, a whopping one hundred thousand times the earth's background magnetic field.

Then we have magnets "As Seen on TV." These cute little magnets fit in bracelets or belts or are sewn into pillows. They're supposed to heal your low back sprain/strain or relieve the pain of degenerative arthritis of the spine. Incidentally, the manufacturers also tell you not to use these magnets if you have a pacemaker, an insulin pump, any kind of transdermal drug delivery system, or if you're pregnant, and that's good advice. Some manufacturers say that these magnets can generate fields that are about five hundred to a thousand times the earth's background magnetic field. This means that they may theoretically generate a magnetic field that's 5 percent as powerful as the magnet in the weakest MRI scanner. Do you really believe that one of these magnet belts or pillows is going to have an effect on the tissues 6 inches (15 centimeters) below the surface of the skin of the back? Neither do I.

Acupuncture

I'm actually a fan of acupuncture. I've never seen it used, and I've never had it performed on myself. But physicians whom I respect have seen it used in certain special situations with spectacular results. In fact, one orthopaedic surgeon whom I know very well related the following story to me. A patient had major shoulder reconstructive surgery at a world-famous teaching hospital of a premier American medical school and had acupuncture as his only anesthesia. The patient was comfortable and pain-free throughout the procedure and did well postoperatively.

But that's not the same as using acupuncture to try to relieve the pain of advanced degenerative disc disease, degenerative arthritis, or nerve root irritation. These are all specific anatomic abnormalities involving objective changes to certain structures. Acupuncture may relieve pain for certain conditions, but it cannot cause anatomic abnormalities to change, improve, or regress. At most, it may give some very temporary relief. In my experience examining patients who had acupuncture, I was seeing them because it hadn't worked. Now, admittedly, I was seeing a skewed sample of patients: those who had not had relief from acupuncture treatments. I didn't get to see patients who had acupuncture treatments and said they'd gotten better because, after all, why would they need any further treatment? Unfortunately, I think acupuncture for the relief of lower back pain has to be considered in the same category as the placebo TENS unit and the plastic needle cap placed against the skin: If the patient is well motivated, there's a strong psychological desire to get better as the result of the use of a special technique.

Whirlpool

There's a full moon. There isn't a cloud in the sky, and a million stars are twinkling. You and some friends slip into your hot tub and enjoy the hot, frothing water, feeling oh, so relaxed. Believe me, I hope you enjoy every second. But don't think you're curing your back pain!

The hot bubbling water will have some effect. Remember, moist heat penetrates to a depth of about 1 inch (2 centimeters) below the surface of the skin. But the paraspinal muscles, the facets, and the nerve roots may be 2 to 5 inches (6 to 10 centimeters) deep to the skin—and deeper in obese people. So the heated water itself will have a mild relaxing effect. All those bubbles bombarding the skin may act as a very mild massage.

But be careful! If you're in a hot tub or a whirlpool bath, and you decide to position yourself so that you're immediately adjacent to a water jet that you can direct precisely to a sore spot, and you keep it directed to that spot for ten or twenty minutes, you'll actually make your back pain worse. The barrage will cause irritation rather than relaxation, and the muscle may even go into spasm, which is precisely what you don't want. If you simply go into a swimming pool and stand around or float either on your back or stomach, you'll get just as much benefit as you will from a whirlpool.

Over-the-Counter Aids for the Relief of Back Pain

If you go to your local drugstore, you'll find shelves stocked with things that are supposed to relieve or take away back pain. Unfortunately, they really don't. Let's look at some of them.

INFRARED MASSAGER

This is supposed to combine the two medically proven ingredients of heat and massage. Infrared heat penetrates to a depth of 1 to 1.3 inches (2.5 to 3.5 centimeters), not nearly far enough to affect back muscles and ligaments. And the handheld massager will nicely vibrate the skin but won't really do anything to the paraspinal muscles.

BACK WRAP WITH MICROWAVEABLE HEAT PACK

These come in several varieties. Some are simply placed on the back; others are wrapped around. All use dry heat, and, as you've seen, dry heat penetrates only to a depth of 2 to 3 millimeters. This means it doesn't even penetrate the fatty tissue (subcutaneous tissue) under the skin.

ELECTRIC HEATING PADS

Some of these even have ergonomic controls, which means that the on/off switch is easy to use. The big danger with dry heat from an electric heating pad is not that it barely penetrates the skin. The big danger is that, even if you set it on low heat, if you lie on it so it's between your back and, say, the bed or the sofa and you fall asleep, you can get burned. You can even get a second- or third-degree burn if you leave it on and lie on it overnight.

MEDICATED PAIN RELIEF PATCHES

On the drugstore shelf you can find a self-sticking pad containing LANOLIN! (as the package exclaims) GLUCOSAMINE! and CHONDROITIN! Those three ingredients are prominently listed on the fronts of packages. Turn the packages over and you find that they're there because a topical anesthetic (something that numbs the skin) will dry the skin, and their job is to moisturize it and make it soft. Oh yes, the topical anesthetic, which is the main ingredient? Menthol! What is menthol? It's basically peppermint and is extracted from peppermint oil. When applied to the skin, it does several things. First, it makes capillaries dilate near the skin's surface, and that tends to make heat radiate out through the skin. Second, it triggers the tiny skin nerve endings that sense cold, but it doesn't actually change the skin temperature. Triggering those **cold thermoreceptors** adds to the feeling of coolness. It is the creation of this feeling of coolness that acts like a local anesthetic (remember how putting ice on the skin will make it feel numb). Unfortunately, the effect of the menthol in a pain relief patch is very localized, it's only close to the skin surface, and it has no effect on the back muscles, ligaments, or joints. 'Nuf said.

ELASTIC WORK BELTS AND LUMBAR SUPPORTS

I discussed these in chapter 5, but it's worth repeating here: Over-the-counter elasticized belts, regardless of their width, and wide work belts that close in the front (usually with Velcro) and have over-the-shoulder straps to help keep them positioned do not prevent back pain and do not relieve it. They may serve as a reminder that you should bend, lift, and carry properly, but they won't reduce the chances of developing a low back strain/sprain, herniating a disc, or what have you.

EPSOM SALTS

I've always told my patients that the only thing Epsom salts do is keep the companies that make them in business. Did you know that Epsom salts—magnesium sulfate—is not used in hospitals for soaking? That's because it doesn't have any real therapeutic value as a soaking agent; it's no better than soaking in saline (salt water). That's why hospitals use saline instead of Epsom salts . . . and it's a lot cheaper!

Surface Electromyograms (EMGs)/ Pain Scans

You may see advertisements for, or have a health care provider recommend performing on you, a surface electromyogram, also called a pain scan. This is supposed to be a computerized picture of the spine showing areas that are, well, painful. There are several reasons why you should politely decline.

- ✦ First, pain is a subjective complaint: The patient says that something hurts. We actually have no way of knowing with certainty that this something hurts. In fact, there is no way to test for and quantify pain. The theory behind the surface EMG or pain scan is that electrode patches, similar to those used when you have an electrocardiogram, will pick up the electrical activity in muscles and create a computerized picture that purports to show where the pain is located.

- ✦ Second, although the computer-generated charts and graphs that the surface EMG device creates do look impressive, they are nothing compared to the printout of the health care provider's income statement showing the fee this test generates.

✦ Third, don't take my word for it. Read what the Therapeutics and Technology Assessment Committee of the American Academy of Neurology has to say about surface EMGs (SEMG). Neurologists are medical doctors who have had at least three years of residency after medical school to learn how to diagnose and treat neurologic conditions of the brain, spinal cord, nerve roots, and peripheral nerves.

The subcommittee's report, "Clinical Utility of Surface EMG," was published in the peer-reviewed medical journal *Neurology*. The subcommittee reviewed more than twenty-five hundred original articles, reviews, and books ". . . to determine the scope of SEMG utility, its benefits and risks, and the extent to which SEMG techniques vary, and to assess SEMG's strengths and weaknesses for specific clinical applications."

In its report, the subcommittee defined the purpose of SEMGs: ". . . The presumed association between lower back pain and muscle fatigue provides the rationale for studying pain with SEMG. Nevertheless, the actual association between pain and fatigue has been difficult to establish."

After discussing many studies, the report concluded that ". . . several considerations make the reported SEMG findings in lower back pain of doubtful clinical value. First, although muscle fatigue is thought to be related to the development of lower back pain and is associated with changes in SEMG spectral frequency, the relationship between the two is uncertain. Second, it is unclear what other factors may influence spectral frequency, making the specificity of the SEMG findings in this clinical setting unclear. Third, many of the reports use discriminant functions based on case-control studies, which have not been verified on independent samples of patients and control subjects. Fourth, the actual discriminant functions used have differed between reports."

I saved the best for last: The subcommittee's final conclusion regarding the use of SEMGs in the assessment of lower back pain was, ". . . Fifth and finally, even if the reports are accepted at face value, the findings suggest only that SEMG can identify patients who have lower back pain. Presumably, the gold standard is the clinical history and, in this circumstance, it would be easier and cheaper simply to ask the patient whether his or her back hurts. . . ." I couldn't have said it better myself.

Traction

The theory behind traction is that it will stretch the paraspinal muscles and also distract, or pull apart, the intervertebral disc spaces. In olden times (that is, just thirty years ago!), traction was frequently used in the form of a belt or harness placed around the waist, with straps going down toward the legs. Weights were attached to these straps and then hung over the end of the bed. This kind of traction turned out to be useless because the weight was insufficient and had no effect on the disc spaces.

For one intervertebral disc space to be distracted, it needs to have a force applied to it equal to one-half the body's weight. But when the body is placed in traction, *all* of the disc spaces in the lumbar region are affected. Traction also keeps the patient immobilized for a prolonged period of time, and that can lead to other complications such as deep vein thrombosis.

Another type of traction is **autotraction**, which is made by a variety of manufacturers and can create an amount of pull equal to half the body's weight. But this traction force will be applied to all the intervertebral disc spaces in the lumbar spine, not just the one that's the culprit. Additionally, the various ligaments and the annuli fibrosi of all of the lumbar discs will all absorb and use up a good deal of that traction effort, leaving an insufficient amount of force to be applied to the injured interspace. For traction to be effective, it would have to be applied for at least eight hours at a time. Don't forget: The moment you sit up or stand, all those interspaces that were theoretically just distracted for many hours will instantly compress again as the weight of the upper half of your body pushes down against them.

It's important to note that the traction I've been discussing is unrelated to the traction that's used to immobilize a broken arm or leg or that's used to stabilize an injured neck. The arm, leg, and neck bones can be distracted by ten to forty pounds of traction.

Now that you've learned about the treatments and remedies that really don't work, if you see a doctor for treatment of lower back pain and he tells you to use any of the things I've just described, there are two things I suggest that you do:

1. Show him this chapter and discuss it.

2. Get a second opinion.

Chapter Eight

BACK PAIN DURING PREGNANCY AND AFTER DELIVERY

You're going to have a baby! How wonderful! You have my warmest good wishes for both you and your future baby. You have a special glow about you that you've never had before. You have special warm feelings that you've never experienced before. Of course, if you've had a prior pregnancy, you undoubtedly recall that glow and those feelings. Your skin has a special softness and smoothness that you'd like to bottle and keep with you for the rest of your life.

Unfortunately, you also have a very high chance of developing back pain during your pregnancy. In fact, up to 80 percent of pregnant women can expect to have at least one episode of back pain during pregnancy. This might occur as a single episode associated with one event one time, mild pain that seems to come on with certain activities, or chronic back pain that may continue long after pregnancy.

If you had one or more episodes of back pain before you became pregnant, you have a much higher chance of developing back pain during pregnancy than an expectant mother who's never previously experienced back pain. In addition, if you had back pain before you became pregnant, it's very likely that if you do develop back pain during pregnancy, it will begin earlier than it would in an expectant mother who never had back pain before. Back pain in pregnancy can begin as early as eight to twelve weeks, but most pregnancy-related back pain begins between the fifth and seventh months.

If you have back pain that lasts for several weeks or months during your pregnancy, it may be an indication that you're going to have postpartum (after delivery) back pain. It is also more likely that your postpartum back pain may continue for months and become chronic. Fortunately, the vast majority of pregnant women with back pain will have resolution of their symptoms by about two months after delivery. If your symptoms are not subsiding by that time, it's essential that you be examined and vigorously treated to try to avoid developing chronic lower back pain.

How can such a glorious event become clouded by unpleasant problems? There are four reasons that back pain occurs during pregnancy:

+ **Weight gain.** You'll recall from the section on degenerative arthritis in chapter 4 that lifting with the outstretched hand produces a force of 15 pounds per square inch at the lower lumbar discs. When you gain weight during your pregnancy, you may easily gain an amount equal to 25 percent of your normal body weight. This additional weight creates direct pressure on the lower lumbar spine and sacroiliac joints and increases the amount of work they have to do.

  When you've gained 30 or 35 pounds during your pregnancy, that's really the same as if you were at your pre-pregnant weight but were carrying around a 30- or 35-pound sack of concrete all day. Do you think your back would get sore if you did that all day, every day? Of course, this doesn't mean that you should avoid weight gain during pregnancy! It's just to give you an idea of why you're getting sore. Later on, I'm going to give you a bunch of handy hints to try to avoid that soreness.

+ **A change in your center of gravity.** You learned in chapter 1 that looking at the spine from the side reveals three curves from the neck to the sacrum: a cervical lordotic curve (a C-shaped curve that faces toward the front of the body), a thoracic kyphotic curve (a C-shaped curve that faces toward the back of the body), and a lumbar lordotic curve, just like the cervical one. The effect of these three curves is to keep the body aligned and allow the weight of the upper part of the body to pass downward just slightly in front of the spine. This is called the **weight-bearing line. (Fig. 8–1)** The paraspinal muscles have an easy time maintaining this posture; in fact, you can be erect all day and never give a second thought to what your body's doing.

Figure 8-1

Weight-Bearing Line

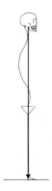

In the second and third trimesters of your pregnancy, however, your growing baby adds extra weight in front of the normal weight-bearing line and shifts your center of gravity forward. If you did nothing, that extra weight in front of you would tend to pull you so far forward that you'd just about tip over. Your body tries to prevent that from happening by having you stand with more extension in your lumbar spine: You begin to assume a swayback posture with excessive lumbar lordosis. By doing this, you shift the weight-bearing line back to where it

belongs; you restore your center of gravity to its proper location and avoid being tipped forward. This excessive lordotic
posture, unfortunately, can make for a very nagging backache.

✦ **Stretched abdominal muscles.** As your baby develops inside
you, your uterus enlarges. As it enlarges, it stretches the front
of the abdominal cavity so that it can be properly accommo-
dated. But stretching the abdominal cavity means stretching
the abdominal muscles in the front and sides. The front abdominal muscle is called the **rectus abdominis**. (That's Latin
for the straightener of the stomach.) The side abdominal muscles are called the **internal** and **external obliques** and **transverse abdominals**.

In chapter 1, you learned that the abdominal muscles are responsible for pulling you forward (flexing the spine). In chapter
5, you learned some exercises to strengthen them because they
can help unload the spine and make its work easier. They can't
function well when they're stretched, so the lower back has to
work harder, and you may suffer as a result. Later in this chapter, I'm going to review those exercises and add others.

✦ **Relaxing hormones of pregnancy.** You don't need a degree in
mechanical engineering to understand that the diameter at the
shoulders of a full-term baby is too big for the lower pelvis
through which it's supposed to travel. Your body knows this, and
does something special to help: It makes a special hormone
called **relaxin**, which has the property of causing ligaments
and muscles to—you guessed it!—relax. During pregnancy, the
concentration of relaxin in the bloodstream becomes ten times
as high as it is in a nonpregnant woman.

Remember those dense, thick, tough, unyielding sacroiliac ligaments I talked about in chapter 5? Well, they become pussy-
cats in the presence of relaxin and, in late pregnancy, they *do*
relax and allow the sacroiliac joints to open up kind of like a

hinge. This widens the pelvis and allows vaginal childbirth to occur. But as the sacroiliac ligaments relax and this opening up gradually occurs, you may develop the very same kind of pain as the patient with the sacroiliac strain in chapter 5. The effect of relaxin on the sacroiliac joints in late pregnancy is also responsible for the waddling type of gait that many women develop then. Later in this chapter, you'll see what can be done to try to ease that discomfort.

The back pain that's associated with pregnancy can be one of two types: **lumbar pain** and **pelvic pain**.

Lumbar pain is basically no different from the pain adults feel when they have a low back muscle strain. It's related to prolonged sitting, to standing or walking, and, of course, to carrying. It's usually found at waist level or just above it, and usually does not include radiating leg pain. Sometimes, however, radiating pain to the leg or foot may become quite prominent. The paraspinal muscles themselves may also be sore.

Pelvic pain is different. It's located at the waistline in the back (posteriorly) and so is also called **posterior pelvic pain**. It goes *down* the back of the pelvis and often includes the sacrum, the sacroiliac joints, and the hip joints. Sometimes it comes around the front of the pelvis to the pubic bones. It may go down the backs of the thighs, but it rarely goes below the knees. It may be on one side (**unilateral**) or on both sides (**bilateral**). It happens to pregnant women *four times as often* as lumbar pain does.

Pelvic pain can occur even in pregnant women who have been exercising regularly prior to pregnancy and who are in good physical condition. It is aggravated by a whole host of things, including lifting, twisting, prolonged sitting, arising from a sitting position, going up and down stairs, walking, running, rolling over in bed, standing at a worktable for a prolonged period of time, and more. Unfortunately, it may not be relieved by rest, which means that it's present even when you're lying down. It also may be accompanied by marked stiffness when you awaken and attempt to get out of bed.

There can also be **obstetric causes of pelvic pain**, and these have absolutely nothing to do with the spine, even if they are accompanied by backache. Two ominous causes of pelvic pain are placental separation and a leaking ovarian cyst. So if your pelvic pain is severe or if it is associated with other signs or symptoms, you should be evaluated *immediately* by your obstetrician.

It's important to keep in mind that back pain should not be thought of as something that you must have or that you will be plagued with it throughout your pregnancy. Yes, you have an excellent chance of having back pain *at some time* during your pregnancy. That doesn't mean that you have to resign yourself to it. If you do, the whole wonderful experience of pregnancy may become unpleasant and complicated by unnecessary extra stress. You may find that, because of your pain, you need to miss work or forgo many activities. Untreated, your back pain may cause added problems not only during delivery, but after it as well.

The best thing, of course, is to try to avoid getting back pain in the first place. There are many things you can do on your own to help reduce your chances of developing lumbar or even posterior pelvic pain. Some are quite simple, take virtually no effort, and can be of great help. Here they are.

Handy Hints for Trying to Avoid Back Pain During Pregnancy

1. Wear shoes that have a good arch support and low heels. Flat shoes and high-heeled shoes are both bad because they cause a shift in the weight-bearing line, the center of gravity, and that makes the back and abdominal muscles have to work harder.

2. If you must stand for prolonged periods, get a little footstool and put one foot on it. The stool doesn't have to be very high, and you should switch feet frequently. Placing one foot on a

stool will cause a change in lordosis and make standing much more comfortable.

3. Stand up straight with your shoulders squared. In other words, try to keep them back a bit, imitating the posture of soldiers.

4. Use proper lifting techniques. That means *not* bending from the waist when you want to pick up something. Instead, bend your knees and lift using your legs, or, if necessary, get down on one knee with the other foot firmly planted, pick up the object, and then rise.

5. Keep the object you're lifting close to your body. Remember, keeping your arms outstretched while lifting causes a large increase in forces on your lower back.

6. Better yet, get someone else to do the lifting for you!

7. Try to avoid having to carry heavy objects. When you shop for groceries, ask for more bags with fewer items in them. When you get home, if the bags are still too heavy, take out a few items at a time to avoid carrying the whole bag at once.

8. If you already have another small child or children, be very careful when lifting them. Use the same techniques listed in tips 4 and 5 above. Better yet, use the technique listed in 6! Also, small children are great helpers and can bend down for you and pick up things especially if you make it a game.

9. If you have to bathe small children, do so by kneeling at the tub. Put some folded towels on the floor to make it more comfortable. Don't bend over at the waist.

10. Sleep on a firm mattress. If yours is too soft, have someone put a bed board (at least 0.6 inch thick—1.5 centimeters) between the mattress and the box spring.

11. Lie on your side in bed, with your knees flexed (bent) and with a pillow between them. My daughter swears by pregnancy pillows—giant pillows that are nearly as long as your body.

12. If you do lie on your back, put a pillow under your knees and calves. You've now assumed the reclining chair posture (the semi-Fowler's position mentioned in chapter 7) and have markedly reduced the pressure on the low back. You may, however, find that you have also markedly reduced your ability to breathe.

13. Sit up straight and use a chair with a high enough back. Sitting posture is very important in maintaining proper alignment and easing the work the muscles have to perform.

14. You may also use a small pillow behind your back when you're sitting. It will help you maintain correct posture and also provide some additional lumbar support.

15. If you must sit for prolonged periods, use a small footstool and alternate placing one foot on it.

16. Swimming is an excellent way to keep your back muscles strong and pain-free while not placing them under excessive stress because of the buoyant effect of the water.

17. Do regular home exercises, which I'll describe later in this chapter.

18. Reduce physical activities. Yeah, I know: That's easy for me to say! But if you can cut down on prolonged standing, walking, stair climbing, and the like, it will go a long way toward helping you avoid back pain.

19. Try to arrange your work schedule so that you can take several breaks during your shift in which you can at least sit with your feet propped up—or, better still, lie down.

20. Use every ergonomic trick there is at your workplace. Understanding the actual mechanics of what you do in your job can be an excellent way to avoid stressing your back.

The proper attitude to take if you do develop back pain during pregnancy is *treat it promptly*. It will do you no good to spend days being miserable, waiting for your pain to go away by magic. You should arrange to see your obstetrician as soon as possible if you develop back pain, regardless of whether it's lumbar or posterior pelvic pain. First and foremost, you want to be certain that it's "only" back pain and not something else.

Your obstetrician may refer you to an orthopaedic surgeon (also called an orthopaedist) for further evaluation and for treatment. Ask to be referred to an orthopaedist who understands and has treated the back pain of pregnancy, both lumbar and posterior pelvic. You'll have a physical examination of your back and legs. You won't have x-rays, however, because they'd be dangerous to your baby. You may be given a series of exercises that you can do at home. You may be referred for a short course of physical therapy. You may be prescribed a special pregnancy back support. Unfortunately, you can't be given prescriptions for any of the medicines that often help relieve back pain because they're not to be used during pregnancy.

Let's look closer at what can be done to ease your back pain and possibly—or probably—get it to clear up completely.

Home Exercises

Ideally, you will have begun a program of home back and abdominal strengthening exercises very early in your pregnancy, before there was even any hint of back pain. These exercises can be invaluable in helping to avoid developing back pain, but you must use common sense!

✦ Before you begin a program of home exercises, you *must* speak to your doctor to make certain that there is no contraindication to your doing them.

✦ They should be done in such a way that there's no weight from your upper abdominal cavity and thorax pressing on your pelvis.

✦ You should not have pain while you're doing these exercises. If you develop abdominal pain—or any other symptoms that seem unusual—*stop immediately and call your doctor!*

✦ If you get pain that radiates down your leg or numbness or paresthesias (pins and needles) in your leg or foot or toes, *stop immediately and call your doctor!*

✦ Do not do weight-bearing exercises. These can cause increased pain and stress the joints.

If you've developed back pain and seen your obstetrician and possibly a specialist, often the first line of defense—and often the *only* treatment that's needed—is a series of home exercises. I've discussed some of them in chapter 5, but I'm going to review them again here so there's no confusion, and then I'm going to add others that are particularly useful during pregnancy.

The first group of exercises should be done only during the first trimester! That's because it's usually not good to lie on your back as your pregnancy progresses. Not only does it become increasingly uncomfortable, but it also can put pressure on blood vessels and other structures as the enlarging uterus presses against the back of the abdominal cavity and the spine.

Supine Flexion

To do this exercise, lie on the floor on your back with your hands at your sides and your knees bent to a comfortable degree. (**Fig. 8–2A**) As you do this exercise, *keep your knees bent at all times; do not straighten your legs.* Hold on to your knees with your hands, (**Fig. 8–2B**) and pull your knees toward your chest as far as you can. (**Fig. 8–C**) Hold this position for several seconds and then slowly return to the resting position. *Keep the back of your head on the floor and do not raise your head while you do this exercise.* You can repeat this exercise twenty to thirty times, and you can do it two, three, or four times a day.

Figure 8-2

Supine Flexion

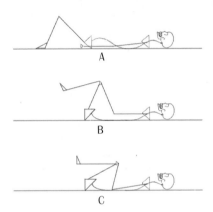

A

B

C

Sacroiliac Stretching

Sacroiliac stretching is done lying on the floor on your back with your legs out straight. Ideally you should have someone push down on the bony bump that's located in line with your belly button but at the front side of the pelvic bone (the ilium) just above the hip joint on the same side as the sore sacroiliac joint (which, of course, is on the back side of the pelvis). (**Fig. 8–3A**) This bump is called the anterior superior iliac spine or ASIS. While the ASIS is being pushed down, either swing that leg with the knee straight across the other leg as far as possible and hold for about five seconds, (**Fig. 8–3B**) or bend the knee of that leg and try to get that knee across the other leg and pointing down toward the floor for about five seconds. (**Fig. 8–3C**) It isn't easy, but with practice you'll get the hang of it. Repeat it ten to twenty times and do it two or three times daily.

Sacroiliac Stretching

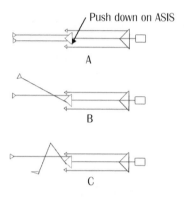

Unfortunately, this should only be done during the first trimester, so you won't be able to do it if you're getting sacroiliac discomfort during the third trimester when the relaxin hormone is doing its job.

PELVIC TILTS

Pelvic tilts are done while lying on your back with your knees flexed (bent) and your feet flat on the floor. (**Fig. 8–4A**) Tighten the muscles of your stomach and buttocks, tilt your pelvis backward, and push your low back against the floor. (**Fig. 8–4B**) Hold this position for a second or two, then relax for several seconds. You can repeat this exercises ten times, gradually building to twenty times, and you can do it two or three times daily.

SUPINE COMBINED ARM AND LEG EXTENSION

Supine combined arm and leg extension is done while you lie on your back. As you do this exercise, keep your back and torso flat and try not to move them. Raise your straight *right arm* and your straight *left leg* at the same time. The leg should be lifted 10 to 20 inches (25 to 50 centimeters) above the floor. (**Fig. 8–5A**) Hold this position for about five seconds, then relax. Then do the same thing with the opposite extremities, the *left arm* and *right leg*. (**Fig. 8–5B**) Repeat this ten to fifteen times.

Figure 8-4

Pelvic Tilts

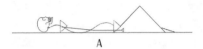

A

Tilt pelvis backward

B

Figure 8-5

Supine Combined Arm and Leg Extension

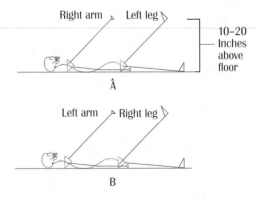

Right arm   Left leg

10–20 Inches above floor

Â

Left arm   Right leg

B

MINI SIT-UPS

Mini sit-ups are an excellent abdominal exercise and work on the rectus abdominis, the center part of the abdominal muscles. Lie on your back with your knees bent. **(Fig. 8–6A)** Lift your head and thorax about 6 inches (15 centimeters) off the floor and hold for a second, then relax. **(Fig. 8–6B)** *Do not* put your hands *behind* your head and then pull up your head to do this exercise! That's a sure way to hurt your neck. Instead, place your palms, with fingers together or apart, on the sides of your head at your eyes, as if your hands were blinders on a horse. That way, you can't put pressure on the back of your neck. Start out doing this exercise ten times, then gradually increase so that you can do twenty or thirty. Do this exercise twice a day.

Figure 8-6

Mini Sit-Ups

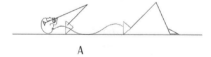

A

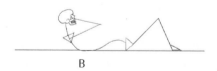

B

BICYCLE MINI SIT-UPS

The bicycle mini sit-up is a fancier version of the above exercise for those who are already in fairly good shape. It's also done while you're lying on your back on the floor. As you lift your head and thorax off the floor in this exercise, with your hands at the sides of your face and your elbows pointing toward your knees, try to bring the *left* elbow to the *right* knee, (**Fig. 8–7A**) then the *right* elbow to the *left* knee. (**Fig. 8–7B**) Again, start out doing ten of each, and gradually build up to twenty or thirty. Do this twice a day. Remember my earlier discussion of the various abdominal muscles, including the internal and external obliques? Well, this exercise works on the obliques. You can only do it during the first trimester; if you are able to do it, this exercise and the one above may help a lot later on in your pregnancy because your abdominal muscles will be better able to provide support.

Figure 8-7

Bicycle Mini Sit-Ups

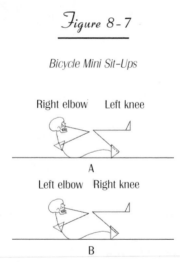

Right elbow   Left knee

A

Left elbow   Right knee

B

BICYCLE WITHOUT THE MINI SIT-UPS

Bicycle without the mini sit-ups is also done while you're lying on your back on the floor. Keep your arms at your sides. Do not raise your head; perform just the bicycling maneuver with your legs, alternating bringing your left and right knees toward your chest. (**Fig. 8–8A,B**)

Start out doing ten and gradually build up to twenty or thirty. Do this twice a day.

Figure 8-8

Bicycle

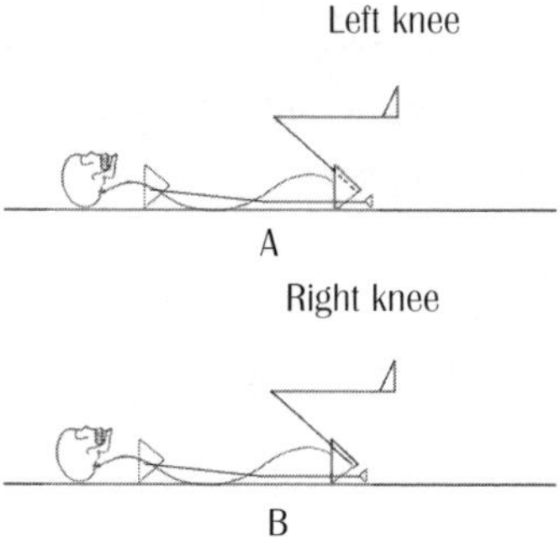

Left knee

A

Right knee

B

The next group of exercises may be done throughout your pregnancy.

SITTING FLEXION

Sitting flexion will do the opposite of the extension exercises above. Sit on a firm chair or stool with your legs apart (forming a V) and your hands resting on your knees. (**Fig. 8–9A**) Bend forward slowly at the waist, touching the floor with your hands. (**Fig. 8–9B**) Hold this position for several seconds, then slowly return to the sitting position. You can repeat this exercise twenty to thirty times, and you can do it two, three, or four times a day. There may come a point in your pregnancy when this exercise starts to become too uncomfortable. Don't do it then!

SITTING FLEXION TO EXTENSION

Sitting flexion to extension is very easy to do. Sit on a firm chair or stool with your legs in front of you. Sit in a very slouched position for several seconds. (**Fig. 8–10A**) Then slowly straighten up and make your back as extended as possible—the other extreme—with a nice hollow in it. (**Fig. 8–10B**) Hold this for several seconds, then return to the first position. It's important to do this slowly and smoothly, without any jerky movements. You can repeat this exercise twenty to thirty times, and you can do it two, three, or four times a day. This exercise is really good if you have back pain and must continue to work at a job that involves prolonged sitting.

Figure 8-9

Sitting Flexion

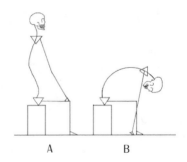

A   B

Figure 8-10

Sitting Flexion to Extension

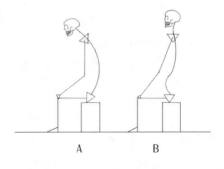

A   B

STANDING PELVIC TILTS

Standing pelvic tilts are done by standing with your back against a wall, legs straight, and feet together. **(Fig. 8–11A)** Tilt your pelvis upward as you flatten your lower back against the wall. **(Fig. 8–11B)** Hold this position for a second or two, then relax for several seconds. You can repeat this exercise ten times, and gradually build to twenty times, and you can do it two or three times daily.

Figure 8-11

Standing Pelvic Tilts

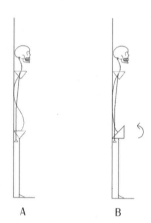

A   B

SIDE-LYING PELVIC TILTS

Side-lying pelvic tilts are done—you guessed it—while you lie on your side either on the floor or on your bed. You can flex your knees (and even put a pillow between them), **(Fig. 8–12A)** then tilt your pelvis backward as you attempt to straighten your low back against an imaginary wall. **(Fig. 8–12B)** Hold this position for a second or two, then relax for several seconds. You can repeat this exercise ten times and gradually build to twenty times, and you can do it two or three times daily.

Figure 8-12

Side-Lying Pelvic Tilts

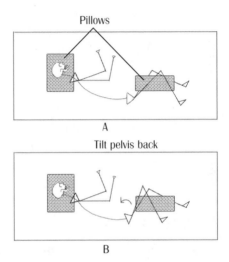

Pillows

A

Tilt pelvis back

B

SIDE-LYING LEG LIFTS

Side-lying leg lifts are also done while you lie on your side on the floor. Keep both legs straight. You can either prop your head on your hand or side-lie with your head on a pillow. (**Fig. 8–13A**) Tighten the thigh muscles and the buttock muscles, then lift your straight leg about 10 inches (25 centimeters) off the floor. (**Fig. 8–13B**) It's important to keep the kneecap of that leg facing straight forward at all times. Otherwise, if you turn your leg outward a bit, so that the kneecap starts pointing upward, you've changed the alignment and pull of the muscles; then the exercise is much less effective. Hold this position for three to five seconds, bring the leg back down slowly, and rest for several seconds. Repeat ten times. Roll over and do the same exercise for the other leg. You can do this two or three times daily.

Figure 8-13

Side-Lying Leg Lifts

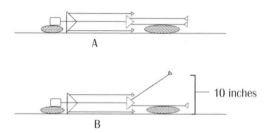

PRONE COMBINED ARM AND LEG EXTENSION

Prone combined arm and leg extension is a nifty exercise that requires just a little bit extra concentration. Position yourself on your hands and knees as if you were going to play "horsie" with a child. Now lift your *right arm* out straight at head height, while *simultaneously* lifting your *left leg* and straightening it. You want to raise the leg as high as you can, but no higher than your hips. (**Fig. 8–14A**) Hold this position for one or two seconds, then relax and do the same thing with the opposite pair of extremities, the *left arm* and the *right leg*. (**Fig. 8–14B**) This is a good exercise for strengthening the abdominal, buttock, and even the shoulder muscles. Repeat it ten or fifteen times and do it two or three times daily.

PRONE BACK ARCH

Prone back arch is also a good exercise for the abdominal and back muscles. Did you ever see a cartoon where a cat is angry and has really arched its back? Well, that's what you're going to try to re-create . . . without the anger. Get on your hands and knees in the "horsie" position, with your arms going straight down below, and not in front of, your shoulders, and your thighs going straight down as well. (**Fig. 8–15A**) Take in a deep breath; as you let it out, arch your back like the angry cat, and make it as arched as possible. (**Fig. 8–15B**) Hold it for several seconds, then relax. Do ten to fifteen of these and repeat two or three times daily. By the way, according to my daughter, once you get into position for this exercise, you will never want to get up. When you let your uterus hang away from your body, you'll be able to fill your lungs with air—something that's very difficult to do when your baby and your expanded uterus are taking up all the space in your abdominal cavity.

Figure 8-14

Prone Combined Arm and Leg Extension

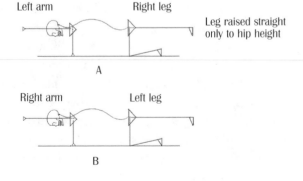

Figure 8-15

Prone Back Arch

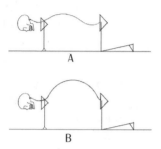

A

B

Physical Therapy

If home exercises alone don't take away your back pain, then you may be sent for a course of physical therapy. If this happens, you should ask your doctor to be referred to a therapist who has a lot of experience in dealing with pregnant women, because not all do—and there are specialized techniques to be employed . . . and sometimes to be avoided.

The only modalities that can be safely used are moist heat and ice. Remember, moist heat penetrates to a depth of about 1 inch (2.5 centimeters) below the surface of the skin. It won't have any effect on the uterus or baby. Ice, when used for short periods, likewise will have no effect. It's an entirely different story with ultrasound and microdyne: They're designed to heat deep structures up to 7 inches (17.5 centimeters) below the skin's surface. They *can* cause injury to the uterus and baby and should never be used during pregnancy. Deep friction massage is also a no-no. But gentle back massage, gentle soft-tissue mobilization techniques, joint mobilization, gentle stabilization techniques, stretching exercises, and certain strengthening exercises will all help.

The therapist will also go over with you in detail how you maintain correct posture, how you utilize proper body mechanics in performing activities of daily living, home exercises, and will analyze your work activities, and so on. Another important part of physical therapy will be instructions on techniques for easing your back pain during labor and delivery.

If your problem can be successfully treated, most of the time you only need anywhere from two to six sessions with the therapist. If your symptoms persist, the therapist—and this should *always* be in direct consultation with your obstetrician and orthopaedist, if you were referred to one—may recommend the use of a specially designed back support for pregnant women. There are several types, including back braces, elastic slings, nonelastic binders, and maternity girdles.

Very rarely, your back pain and accompanying leg symptoms may be due to a herniated disc. That's not good. The first inclination of the patient, and often of the doctors who are treating her, is to try to do everything to avoid surgery, at least until sometime after delivery. But that won't always be the right thing to do, especially if the symptoms are accompanied by physical examination findings and electromyogram and nerve conduction test results that clearly confirm signs of nerve root irritation. Of course, you won't be able to have a CAT scan, an MRI scan, a myelogram, or a discogram to make easy work of the diagnosis, but a careful physical examination plus EMGs and NCTs will provide all the information that's needed in this case. Unremitting pain, numbness and paresthesias (pins and needles), along with unequivocal signs of marked nerve root pressure really should not wait for proper treatment. And the proper treatment is surgery.

In the olden days, thirty years ago, if you had lumbar disc surgery, you were placed facedown on an operating table and the table was then "jackknifed" so it looked like this: ^. We've made great strides since then. Now patients are positioned on a heavily padded frame so that they are in a kneeling position, the entire abdomen is hanging free and not touching anything, and the chest is well supported. That's safe for the baby. The anesthetics that are used are also safe for the baby. If you wait until some time after delivery to have surgery, you run the risk of ending up with permanent nerve root damage, which means permanent changes in the muscles and skin the nerve root supplies. I don't think that's a smart thing to do.

If your back pain during your pregnancy is not from a herniated disc but from one of the other causes I've discussed, and if it continues after you've delivered, then several things can be done. If it was lumbar pain, all the things that can be done for a low back strain (see chapter 5 for the details) can be started beginning several weeks postpartum. If it's persistent posterior pelvic pain—especially persistent sacroiliac joint pain—then this is a good time to begin using a sacroiliac belt for compression. The other forms of treatment that were described in chapter 5 can also be employed.

Finally, there's one more kind of back pain that you may develop late in your pregnancy that I haven't discussed yet. It's called labor pain and, I'm told, is like severe menstrual cramping. It's unremitting, meaning it doesn't go away, it's unrelated to activities, and it gets stronger and stronger (patients would probably say "worse and worse") in a relatively short time.

If you're experiencing this specific kind of pain while you're reading this, please do me a favor: Stop reading. Put this book down. Grab your previously packed suitcase. Go quickly to the hospital because *you're having a baby!* Good luck!

Chapter Nine

OUR BACKS AS WE AGE

Did you watch snowboarders at the most recent Winter Olympics or gymnasts at the last Summer Olympics? Have you seen commercials on TV where young male and female rock stars gyrate as they sing? Have you watched college football and basketball players twist, jump, leap, get knocked down . . . and bounce right back up? And then have you thought, *How come I can't do that stuff anymore? And if I try to do it, how come my back gets as stiff as a board?* There's a very simple but sobering answer to these questions: You're older than they are, and your body has aged.

How Vertebrae Develop and Grow

You learned about the appearances and consequences of aging in chapters 4 and 6. But you need to understand how and why these things happen. To do this, you'll need to learn a little about how vertebrae form, grow, and age. I've hinted at some of these things in the earlier chapters, but now I'm going to tie everything together.

In a developing fetus, the first signs of formation of the structure that will become the spinal column and spinal cord occur between the third and fifth weeks. By six to eight weeks, vertebrae have started to separate (we say **segment**) as special tissue comes together to make the vertebral bodies, the laminae (which are called the **neural arch** during fetal development), the discs, and the beginning of the spinal cord. But at this stage, and continuing for many weeks, the vertebrae aren't made of bone; they're made of cartilage. Other cartilage buds grow from the neural arch and make the transverse processes (the gutters of the spinal house) and the spinous processes (the chimneys).

By the time the fetus is fully formed and is ready to be born, most of this cartilage has changed to bone—but not *all* of it. So at birth, the body of the vertebra features a bony center surrounded by cartilage (with an intervertebral disc at each end), and each lamina has a bony center also surrounded by cartilage. But the rest of the vertebra, including the pedicles, is all cartilage. (**Fig. 9–1**)

Figure 9-1

Vertebra of a Newborn

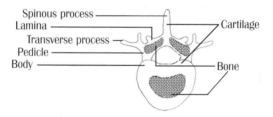

During the first year of life, the two laminae that make one neural arch completely turn to bone and fuse together. During the third to sixth years of life, the bony neural arch fuses to the vertebral body as the cartilaginous parts in between—the pedicles—turn to bone. (**Fig. 9–2**) This process begins in the lumbar spine and progresses upward toward the thoracic and cervical spine. The delay in the fusing of the neural arch to the vertebral body allows the spinal canal to enlarge easily and the spinal cord inside it to grow during those early years. The growth of the spinal canal is rapid during the first five years. During the next five years when the pedicles and neural arch are all bony, the growth slows as the bone itself grows.

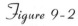

Figure 9-2

Vertebra of a Five-Year-Old

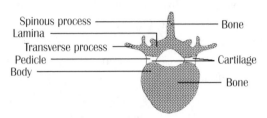

Spinous process — Bone
Lamina
Transverse process
Pedicle — Cartilage
Body — Bone

The spinal canal reaches its final size before the overall growth of the spinal column is completed. The final length of the spine is reached in most girls between the ages of eleven and thirteen; in boys it doesn't occur until age fourteen to sixteen on average. Prior to puberty, the spinous processes and transverse processes are still cartilage. There's also growth cartilage in each vertebral end plate (the flat surfaces of the ends of the bodies of the vertebrae, which abut against the intervertebral discs).

At puberty, bone starts to form in the spinous process, the transverse processes, and the growth cartilage at the vertebral end plates. Some of the cartilage doesn't completely change to bone until age twenty-five! You learned in chapter 1 that some intervertebral discs may begin to lose some of their water of hydration by the age of fifteen or sixteen. In fact, I've seen patients that young whose MRI scans revealed herniated discs, and who had surgery to remove those discs.

What Happens When Vertebrae Develop Abnormally

You can start to understand better how certain conditions occur now that you know some embryology (the study of the developing fetus) and how the vertebral column grows. For instance, if during fetal development, the neural arch of the first sacral vertebra (S_1) manages to separate from the neural arch of S_2, then it will be a distinct, discrete pair of laminae; thus S_1 will be lumbarized and will be a transitional vertebra.

The pedicles should only remain as cartilage until between ages three and six. So what happens if that cartilage doesn't fully change to bone? Bingo! Spondylolysis—the absence of bone in the pars interarticularis (the Scottie dog has a broken neck). And if it happens on both sides of one vertebra, the five- or six-year-old child will have bilateral spondylolysis and will be likely to develop spondylolisthesis (slipping of one vertebra on the next) as he or she grows older.

If the cartilage that makes up one or both of the transverse processes at the fifth lumbar vertebra (L_5) continues to grow instead of turning to bone during puberty, the patient will have developed hemi- or complete sacralization of L_5, and a different form of transitional vertebra will have occurred.

The Balancing Act Between Bone Formation and Bone Destruction

So once the vertebrae have finished growing at age twenty-five, then what? Tissues in the body are constantly being formed and replaced. The easiest example to use is the skin. You constantly shed skin cells every day. You can easily see that if you've had a broken bone that was treated with a cast. When the cast was removed, the skin under the cast was covered with a thick layer of dead cells that never had the opportunity to flake off.

Bone is a living tissue, too, and is constantly being formed and replaced. The cells that make bone are called **osteoblasts** (from the Greek for bone formers), and the cells that break down bone are called **osteoclasts** (from the Greek for bone destroyers).

Bone itself is like a lattice or like the steel columns that hold up a skyscraper; some people also compare it to a honeycomb. The outer part of a bone—the circumferential outer part of a vertebral body, or the inner and outer cortex of a lamina (the two slices of bread in a peanut butter sandwich)—is thick and dense, with the columns spaced very, very closely together. The central part of the bone—the marrow—is much less dense and much more spongy . . . but in a different way from the nucleus pulposus of a disc.

Junior Doctor's Merit Badge Checkpoint

For bone to form, two important ingredients are needed: calcium and vitamin D. But just taking a lot of calcium tablets is not good enough. Calcium can only get from the bloodstream into the bone if vitamin D is also present. That's why milk, a good source of calcium, is fortified with vitamin D.

Another way to get calcium into bones is through weight-bearing exercises—by exercising using weights. It might surprise you to learn that one good exercise that uses weight is walking: You have to propel the weight of your body forward against the force of gravity. Swimming is *not* a weight-bearing exercise because your body is floating and gravity is eliminated. (Swimming *does* build up muscles; it just doesn't do anything for bones.) A certain hormone in women, **estrogen**, is also needed for maintenance of the proper amount of bone content, which we call **bone density**.

Osteoporosis

Up to age thirty, the osteoblasts and the osteoclasts live in harmony with each other, and the amount of bone that's made is equal to the amount that's broken down. After age thirty—yes, you read correctly!—we slowly start to lose bone density: The amount of bone that's broken down, or **resorbed**, slowly starts to exceed the amount of bone that's made, or **formed**. When the amount of bone that's resorbed starts exceeding the amount of bone that's made, that's called **osteoporosis** (from the Greek for bone with holes).

Don't think for a minute that osteoporosis only happens to old people. It can occur in relatively young adults in their thirties and forties. Certainly, when women go through menopause, the lowering of estrogen levels results in an increase of the rate of bone breakdown, or resorption, compared to bone formation, and that lasts for several years. Then the rate of bone loss slows down.

But don't think that osteoporosis only happens to women. It also happens in men, albeit more slowly, because men develop decreasing levels of testosterone at a slower rate than estrogen falls in women. By the time men and women reach the age of sixty-five to seventy, however, bone loss occurs at the same rate in both sexes. In fact, 50 percent of women—that's one out of every two—and 12 percent of men—one out of eight—will have a fracture or broken bone related to osteoporosis. Here's the breakdown:

Age	Men	Women
Up to age 30	The amount of bone that's made equals the amount that's broken down in men and women.	
Ages 30–45	Men and women slowly start to lose bone density, but at different rates.	
Ages 45–55	Men lose bone density more gradually than women do at this age.	As women go through menopause, lower estrogen levels result in a faster rate of bone density loss for several years.
Ages 55–65	Men continue to lose bone density at a gradual pace.	After menopause, women continue to lose bone density, but at a slower rate than before.

Age 65 and over   Bone density loss occurs at the same rate in both sexes. Men and women are now at higher risk for broken bones caused by osteoporosis.

Classic osteoporosis is found in ten million people in the United States, while eighteen million others are at risk for developing it because they've already started to lose bone mass. It's found more commonly in several distinct groups, including white women, Asian women, women who go through menopause early, people who have slender bones, and people who have blood relatives who had osteoporosis.

In the spine, osteoporosis can lead to compression fractures. The loss of bone substance—the destruction of the honeycomb or latticework of the cortex of a vertebral body—results in that vertebral body's being unable to support the weight of the body above it, and it collapses. Usually the collapse is in a wedge shape; occasionally, the whole vertebral body flattens like a pancake.

Another condition that can occur in the osteoporotic vertebral body is called **codfishing**. The osteoporosis weakens the vertebral end plate (the flat surface at the end of the body). The intervertebral disc that abuts against that vertebral end plate then paradoxically becomes relatively tougher and more unyielding than the end plate. The disc then literally starts pushing into the center of the end plate, resulting in a convex appearance of the end plate on a lateral (side-view) x-ray of the spine. (**Fig. 9–3**) Some doctor somewhere decided that this appearance on the lateral x-ray looked like the silhouette of a codfish—hence the name. As you'd expect, the cushioning ability of the disc is nil in this condition, and the flexibility of that part of the spine is also markedly diminished.

What's sobering is the fact that 90 percent of the bone has to be lost or resorbed before we can see that there's been bone loss on a routine x-ray! So you could be undergoing a substantial amount of bone resorption *and not even be aware of it, even if you had an x-ray taken for some other reason.* There is, however, a test that is designed to show evidence of bone loss: dual-energy x-ray absorptiometry, or bone densitometry.

It is especially helpful for women who are premenopausal, menopausal, and postmenopausal. If it is repeated every year or every several years, it can help show the doctor whether you're becoming more osteoporotic and how successful your attempts to increase bone deposition by the use of calcium, vitamin D, weight-bearing exercise, or medications have been.

Figure 9-3

Codfish Vertebra

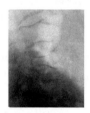

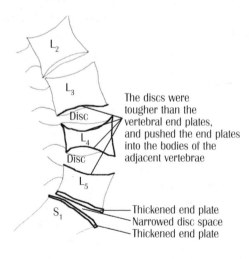

L₂

L₃

Disc

L₄

Disc

L₅

S₁

The discs were tougher than the vertebral end plates, and pushed the end plates into the bodies of the adjacent vertebrae

Thickened end plate
Narrowed disc space
Thickened end plate

X-ray Vision

Codfish vertebrae have very little calcium in them because of the osteoporosis of the patient. That makes the x-ray on page 229 very pale. In fact, this x-ray could barely be seen when photographed, so the black-to-white shades have been inverted to make the vertebrae more visible.

Notice the marked degeneration of the disc between the fifth lumbar and first sacral vertebrae, which we see as tremendous narrowing of the disc space, along with the reaction of the adjacent vertebral end plates, which have greatly thickened.

The Causes—and Results—of Spinal Wear and Tear

You saw in chapters 4 and 6 the other things that can happen during the process of aging, including degenerative disc disease and three forms of osteoarthritis: degenerative arthritis, spinal stenosis, and degenerative spondylolisthesis. These four conditions are all interrelated and are based on the same processes. Many people say that their arthritis must be hereditary because their parents, aunts, uncles, or other relatives had it. But osteoarthritis is a kind of wear-and-tear arthritis, and there's no evidence that it's passed genetically from one generation to the next. The *tendency* toward developing osteoarthritis *may possibly* be genetic, but so far there's no solid proof of this. Instead, arthritis is associated with such lifestyle conditions as being overweight, sports, heavy manual labor, and smoking. Yet it's important to note that some athletes never develop degenerative changes in the spine, while some couch potatoes do.

Junior Doctor's Merit Badge Checkpoint

There is at least one form of arthritis of the spine that may have a hereditary component. It's called **ankylosing spondylitis**, which sounds like a mouthful until you discover that its full name is **Marie-Strumpell rheumatoid ankylosing spondylitis**. It's a special form of rheumatoid arthritis that affects the spinal bones in a unique way: The anterior and posterior longitudinal ligaments turn to bone and fuse the spine as one rigid column. There's a special gene that has a high association with this disease. When this gene is passed on to the next generation, a significant number of people in that generation may develop the disease. Other organs of the body are affected, too. It's beyond the scope of this book, however, and, unfortunately, it can't really be outwitted.

Changes in the Vertebrae and Ligaments

So how do degenerative changes come about in the lumbar spine? The simplest answer is **microtrauma**. You've seen that the vertebral bodies are connected by the anterior and posterior longitudinal ligaments, while the laminae are connected by the ligamentum flavum (the yellow ligament). As we get older, and as bone resorption slowly starts to outpace bone formation, the bone becomes a little bit less able to withstand all the stresses and forces that are applied to it every second that we're up and about, engaging in all of the activities of daily living.

What may happen is that as the ligaments work to keep things properly aligned when these stresses and forces are applied, they're tugging and pulling on the bones to which they attach. Sometimes the extent of this tugging and pulling is such that it exceeds the ability of the bone to keep up, and a tiny, microscopic separation may occur. It's important to keep in mind that even if you could magically look inside the body at the spinal column, you wouldn't be able to see this unless you had a microscope with you. When this microscopic separation occurs, a few blood cells leak out. Again, this microscopic leaking of individual cells is the same as occurs in a muscle sprain, not the kind of bleeding you see when you cut your finger.

For many years, when this occurs, it's not a big deal to the bone, and the blood cells are quickly cleaned up or reabsorbed. But eventually, it does become a big deal to the body, and instead of cleaning up and reabsorbing the leaking blood cells, something else happens. The leaked blood cells turn to bone, so the area where the ligament attached and tugged and pulled becomes a tiny bit thicker. This continues over a period of many months or years, and eventually we can see the formation of a bone spur on an x-ray. The changes are now no longer microscopic.

Many of the bone spurs visible on a lumbar spine x-ray have nothing to do with the normal function of the spine. They're located at the edges of the vertebral bodies as seen on a front-view (**Fig. 9–4**) or side-view (**Fig. 9–5**) x-ray. They represent areas where the longitudinal ligament attachments have turned to bone, and they serve as a visual signal that the spine has become less flexible. Their presence means that the patient isn't going to be doing gymnastics anymore.

The same stresses and forces that I've been discussing also are applied to the ligamentum flavum and laminae. As a result, the ligamentum flavum may start to thicken, and the laminae to which it attaches may do so, as well. Or it could be the other way around: The laminae may begin to thicken as a result of those stresses and forces that are being constantly applied by the paraspinal muscles that attach to them, and *this* may cause the ligamentum flavum, in turn, to thicken. It doesn't really matter which leads to which; what matters is that the thickening that occurs does so both upward (posteriorly, toward the muscles) and downward (anteriorly, toward the spinal canal).

Figure 9-4

X-ray Showing Vertebral Body Spurs

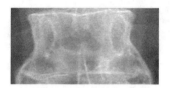

Front view

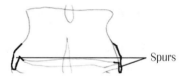

Spurs

X-ray Vision

I chose a rather extreme version of vertebral spurring here to show that x-ray appearance can be misleading: these spurs did not interfere with activity.

Figure 9-5

X-ray Showing Vertebral Body Spurs

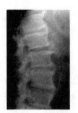

Side view

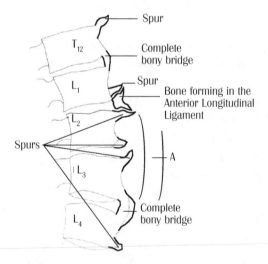

X-ray Vision

This is another example of advanced spur formation. Some of the spurs from adjacent vertebrae have met and fused together, forming a bony bridge. That doesn't cause pain, but it may limit motion slightly.

You may have noticed another structure **(A)** on this side-view x-ray. It's located anterior (in front) to the vertebrae and is, in fact, just inside the abdominal cavity. We can see it because it is full of calcium. You're looking at the calcified walls of the abdominal aorta, the biggest artery in the body. This is classic arteriosclerosis—hardening of the arteries. The diagonal white stripes above it on the x-ray are the ribs.

In addition, these same stresses and forces are transmitted from the laminae down through the pedicles to the vertebral bodies. The pedicles, too, may react to those stresses and forces. As we age, the pedicles may not be able to handle them as efficiently as when we were younger. Extra bone may thus be added—the pedicles thicken—to provide a greater cross section for the forces to be transmitted across. That thickening, however, is also circumferential and narrows not only the spinal canal but also the intervertebral foramen through which the spinal nerve root will exit.

What I've just described is the picture we see as degenerative arthritis occurs in the lumbar spine, and that sometimes progresses all the way to spinal stenosis, two conditions you learned about in chapters 4 and 6. At the same time that all of this is occurring, two other changes may be happening as well.

Changes in the Facet Joints

The first change involves the facet joints. The same stresses and forces get transmitted from one vertebra to the next not only by the anterior and posterior longitudinal ligaments and the ligamentum flavum, but also by the facet joints that literally allow one vertebra to articulate with the next. As we age, sometimes the facet joints can no longer cope with the transmission of the weight of the entire body above them when combined with the additional stresses and forces of work and daily activities. The joint surfaces, including the cartilage and its underlying bone thicken, and the upper part of the facet joint starts sliding on the lower part, causing degenerative spondylolisthesis and often spinal stenosis.

Changes in the Intervertebral Discs

The second change involves the intervertebral discs. You've already learned how the nucleus pulposus (the cherry jelly of the doughnut) can start losing its water of hydration as early as age fifteen or sixteen. The annulus fibrosus (the doughnut) also loses its resilience as the years pass. As you saw earlier, the downward pressure of the weight of the body above the disc causes the aging disc to start to flatten and squish outward. (I compared it to flattening a lump of clay between your palms.) You also learned that the outward-bulging disc pushes up against the anterior and posterior longitudinal ligaments and can eventually result in bone spurs forming.

Discs that bulge can do so in one of several ways: circumferentially, anteriorly, posteriorly, or asymmetrically. All these bulges can be easily seen on either an MRI scan or a CAT scan, on the cross-sectional pictures. (You saw a cross-sectional MRI scan of a bulging disc in chapter 4, figure–4.) A circumferentially bulging disc is usually seen in long-standing advanced degenerative disc disease. An anteriorly bulging disc is unusual by itself, mainly because of the laws of physics: You bend forward much, much more than you bend backward, or extend. As you bend forward, considerable stress is placed on the posterior margin of the disc, forcing it backward. If you spent all day in a posture of extreme lordosis, then anterior-bulging discs would be more common.

A posterior-bulging disc is the most common—and therein lies a kind of danger you wouldn't suspect. The vast majority of posteriorly bulging discs bulge symmetrically from one side to the other. This means that they bulge most prominently in the center, midway between the two pedicles. The most prominent part of the bulge therefore occurs directly below the thecal sac covering the central group of spinal nerve roots as they continue down the spinal canal. (This group of nerve roots is called the **cauda equina**; it continues down below the first lumbar vertebra where the actual spinal cord ends.) A very thin layer of special fatty tissue, called the **epidural fat**, covers the thecal sac circumferentially and acts like a shield on the lower side of it between the thecal sac and the posterior longitudinal ligament.

What's the danger associated with this? Well, let's say you have back pain for whatever reason, and that your doctor sends you for an MRI scan or CAT scan. And let's say the study shows a centrally bulging disc. Unfortunately, many doctors will immediately begin to treat this aggressively, telling you that you may very well need surgery to remove it. Trust me: You don't! A disc that bulges *but does not come into contact with the epidural fat* is no different from a nice, normal, unbulged disc. Since it's not touching the epidural fat, it isn't poking through the epidural fat and thus is not touching the thecal sac. And if it isn't touching the thecal sac, it isn't causing any neurologic symptoms. You'd be surprised by how many doctors don't understand this.

Now, you need to know that normal discs do have a small number of nerve endings, and that these nerve endings are located in the periphery of the annulus fibrosus. Research has shown that as discs degenerate, the number of nerve endings in them increases and may cause disc pain. That's part of the basis for doing a discogram, the x-ray study I described in chapter 2 in which dye is injected into the center of the nucleus pulposus to see if it leaks into the annulus. If fluid is injected under pressure into the disc, the theory is that the disc causing the symptoms will react to the fluid under pressure by causing the same symptoms very intensely. But that's not at all the same as the pain associated with a disc that's pressing on the thecal sac the way a herniated disc does.

An eccentrically bulging disc, the last type of bulge, will be located to either the right or left of the center and may be located between the center and the pedicle, at the level of the pedicle, or beyond the pedicle (referred to as a **lateral bulge**). The same thing applies to this kind of bulge as for the central bulge: If the eccentric bulge isn't touching the thecal sac, it isn't causing any neurologic symptoms.

On the other hand, a lateral bulge that's near the exiting nerve root is sometimes—or often—a different story, because of the relatively narrow space at the intervertebral foramen, the window through which the nerve root exits. A bulge there may well impinge upon or indent the nerve root, and that usually needs surgery. A trial of injections of epidural steroids may help shrink the swelling of the irritated nerve root and reduce or eliminate symptoms. An anesthesiologist who specializes in pain management will use videofluoroscopy to guide a needle down to the foramen next to the nerve root and inject cortisone there. If it works, you've saved yourself an operation . . . possibly permanently.

I can't emphasize strongly enough that doctors should not become slaves to MRI scans and CAT scans, and they should use very jaundiced eyes when looking at what appear to be severe abnormalities. A nifty study performed at George Washington University Medical Center in Washington, DC, showed just what I'm talking about. Sixty-seven male and female patients who had *never* had lower back pain, radiating leg pain, or neurogenic claudication (leg pain when you have spinal stenosis and extend your back) had MRI scans performed on their lumbar spines. The films were read by three different neuroradiologists (doctors whose specialty is reading and interpreting x-ray studies of the nervous system) who knew nothing about the patients.

The neuroradiologists found that, in patients under age sixty, 20 percent had a herniated disc. Over age sixty, 36 percent had a herniated disc and 21 percent had spinal stenosis. In 35 percent of patients between the ages of twenty and thirty-nine, there was at least one bulging or degenerated disc. And there was at least one bulging disc in all but one of the patients between the ages of sixty and eighty. But remember: *Not one of these patients had ever had any symptoms!* What this means, quite simply, is: Just because something abnormal is seen on a special study such as an MRI scan or a CAT scan doesn't mean it has anything to do with anything. Even pathologic abnormalities such as a herniated disc may be completely symptom-free and not need any treatment. What is absolutely crucial is that there be a strict correlation between the findings on the films and the actual symptoms and physical examination of the patient along with the results of any other tests.

Chapter Ten

STAYING OUT OF TROUBLE
PREVENTIVE MAINTENANCE

Now that you've read this far and learned about all the awful things that can happen to your back, you might have become a bit discouraged. You may be thinking, *I'm doomed to have back pain sometime, and there's nothing I can do to stop it!* I can't promise you that you'll never have an episode of back pain. I can't promise you that you'll never develop degenerative arthritis or degenerative disc disease. But I can show you a number of things you can begin doing to minimize the chances of having these things occur—even if you've had multiple episodes of back pain in the past. Some may seem too simple, some may even seem stupid, but all of them have one thing in common: They really help!

As an incentive for you to consider these ideas, I'd like to discuss some things that aren't usually talked about when doctors tell their patients about the need for surgery. Orthopaedic and neurologic surgeons who perform back surgery believe with our whole hearts that we're doing so in order to make our patients better. We believe that, most of the time, we will be able to take away the pain and discomfort our patients have been plagued with and that we'll help restore normal function to their lives. Most of the time, that's exactly what happens, and those patients are some of the happiest people you'd ever want to meet. There are few things as delicious as awakening after back surgery and finding that your previous pain, paresthesias (pins and needles), and numbness are gone. But unfortunately, that doesn't always happen. In fact, some patients continue to experience some degree of pain. A few even occasionally end up worse rather than better.

The Downside of Disc Surgery

Of all the people who develop back pain each year in the United States, only about 2 to 3 percent actually have a herniated disc. That doesn't seem like a lot, until you realize that more than two hundred thousand lumbar laminectomies are performed each year for herniated discs. Various studies have shown that the immediate success rate for this operation can vary from around 50 to 90 percent. Put another way, though, this means that anywhere from 10 to 50 percent of patients having a lumbar laminectomy did *not* improve.

That's not the end of the not-so-good news. After you've had surgery and have fully recovered—even if you're one of the patients who had a perfect surgical result, are 100 percent pain-free, and are doing everything you ever did before your laminectomy—it's possible that degenerative changes may occur in the future. A number of different things can happen.

1. The removal of the nucleus pulposus may result, as years pass, in gradual collapse of that intervertebral disc space. As this occurs, the vertebral end plates will start to thicken, and spurs may develop in the attaching anterior and posterior longitudinal ligaments. This may result in increased stiffness and some loss of motion.

2. If the disc space does narrow, it is also possible that the facet joints associated with that interspace may be affected. The narrowed disc space means that the apposing surfaces of the facet will be pressed more tightly against each other, leading to degenerative arthritic changes—which will then add to the problems associated with degenerative disc disease.

3. The degenerative changes in the facet joints may result in bony thickening, or hypertrophy, of them. This, in turn, may cause narrowing of the adjacent intervertebral foramen, the window through

which the nerve root exits. As a result, there may be radiating leg symptoms of pain, paresthesias (pins and needles), and/or numbness as a consequence of the nerve root irritation.

4. The facet surfaces may also begin to slide, with the upper one sliding down over the lower one, leading to degenerative spondylolisthesis.

5. If the degenerative changes in the interspace occur asymmetrically, and/or the facet arthritis becomes severe enough, a certain degree of instability may also occur. That means that the vertebrae on each side of the degenerated interspace and/or facet no longer work as a smooth unit when they move. The degenerative changes will eventually lead to possible tilting of the vertebra above or to loss of normal gliding motion in the facet—or both—and that is instability. It goes without saying that this is painful.

6. And if these degenerative changes result in extensive bony thickening, or hypertrophy, spinal stenosis may result at that level.

Of course, it's also possible that a new nucleus pulposus will form at the interspace where the surgery was performed and that the new one will function just fine. But remember: In chapter 6, I described a patient who herniated the regenerated nucleus pulposus several years after her initial, successful lumbar laminectomy. Also, sometimes not every last bit of nucleus may be removed at the initial surgery. Later on, a degenerated piece may break off and migrate up against—or through—the posterior longitudinal ligament and result in a recurrent herniated disc.

After a disc has been removed at one level, there is an increase in the forces and stresses at the next-higher intervertebral disc space. Over a period of years, these increased forces can lead to the appearance of degenerative changes at that level, including narrowing of that disc space due to degeneration of the disc, facet joint changes including narrowing and hypertrophy, and vertebral end plate thickening and/or spurring.

As a result of all of these wonderful facts that I've just given you, studies have shown that ten years after having undergone a lumbar laminectomy, up to half of patients will have episodes of severe back

pain. In addition, up to 30 percent will have had severe episodes of radiating leg pain, paresthesias (pins and needles), and numbness. But don't
forget: This also means that more than half will *not* have had severe
back pain, and at least 70 percent will not have had radiating leg symptoms, either.

The Downside of Fusion Surgery

I've talked about lumbar laminectomies; now let's talk about lumbar
spine fusions. In 1986, about seventy thousand spine fusions were performed on the lumbar spine. By 2000, that number had almost doubled
to 130,000. In California alone between 1995 and 1999, there were
92,372 lumbar spine fusion procedures performed. Sixty-five percent of
these were done for degenerative arthritis, facet arthritis, spondylolisthesis, degenerative disc disease, et cetera. The number of anterior
lumbar interbody fusions (where the operation is done through the abdominal cavity and the marrow bone graft is inserted from the front)
increased by more than 200 percent during this period.

Just as certain changes may occur in the adjacent vertebrae after a
lumbar laminectomy, so, too, similar changes may occur after a spine
fusion. There may be hypertrophy of the fused facet joints leading to
narrowing of the intervertebral foramen and pressure on the existing
nerve root. There also may be bone spur formation.

Other changes are unique to lumbar spine fusions. These changes
may occur because the spine fusion alters the dynamics of motion
above the fused levels. In other words, because motion has been taken
away from a portion of the lumbar spine, the vertebrae above the fused
area have to take over to maintain motion and flexibility. These changes
may result in the following problems.

1. There may be degenerative disc disease at the level just above the
    fusion because that level has to become extra mobile. The extra
    mobility may then accelerate wear and tear of the disc.

2. For reasons not at all well understood, after the laminae are solidly fused, their undersurfaces that face the spinal canal may occasionally thicken and cause spinal stenosis.

3. The facet joints at the level above the fusion may become hypertrophic because they have to accommodate extra motion. Degenerative changes can also occur in the facet joints as a result.

4. The instrumentation (metal plates, screws, and so on) may, in very rare instances, become loose during the time it takes for fusion of the graft to occur. This can cause the following changes.

   ✦ The fusion may settle, or collapse, during healing, resulting in a change in alignment. If one side of the fusion settles, there may be asymmetric tilting as a result of the loosening of the instrumentation. (However, the same thing may also happen if no spinal instrumentation was used to help maintain alignment.)

   ✦ There may be pain at the site where the bone graft material was taken from the ilium (the pelvic bone).

   ✦ If an anterior lumbar interbody fusion was performed, occasionally the bone graft that was inserted into the intervertebral disc space may become loose and partially extrude forward. This could result in a poor fusion and need revision. In rare circumstances, it could cause problems with the large blood vessels in front of the spine.

   ✦ If a metal cage with graft material inside it is used, under very rare circumstances it, too, could shift during healing.

One excellent study reviewed patients who had had lumbar spine fusions without instrumentation and who were evaluated anywhere from twenty-one to thirty-three years after their surgery to see how they were doing. Fifteen percent of these patients needed to have a second operation because of problems that had arisen at some point after the first fusion. Almost half of the entire group were taking pain medicine because of back pain. Once again, keep in mind the other side of this story: 85 percent of patients who'd had spine fusions without instrumentation did *not* need repeat surgery, even after thirty-three years had passed since the original procedure, and more than half of all the patients were still pain-free.

Okay, so by now you're probably thinking, *Wow, I'm never going to have surgery, even if I need it! Those complications sound so gruesome that it can't be worth the risk.* You're wrong! It *is* worth it, if you really need surgery, because most people will do well postoperatively, won't have complications, will have excellent long-term results, and won't need repeat surgery. But wouldn't it be nicer if you could do things to try to avoid getting in that situation in the first place? I gave this chapter its title for a reason, and now that you've seen the worst possible outcomes for treatment of back pain, it's time to learn how to keep out of trouble.

What to Do to Keep Your Back Healthy and Avoid Problems

If you do sedentary work, sitting at a desk all day, and if you lead pretty much a couch-potato life the rest of the time, not doing manual labor or sports, you may think that you're immune to developing degenerative arthritis, degenerative disc disease, or spinal stenosis— after all, you don't do anything that really stresses your back muscles, bones, or joints. Not so! In my practice, I saw many patients who lived lives just as I've described here, but whose x-rays showed the very things I listed above. I also saw many athletes as well as people who engaged in vigorous weekend sports activities such as tennis, basketball, or rugby whose x-rays did not show degenerative changes. Why?

WEIGHT

Now, not every thin person has a perfect spine, and not every overweight person has a spine riddled with arthritis. If you read chapter 8, Back Pain During Pregnancy and After Delivery, you'll remember that carrying a third-trimester baby is like walking around all day carrying a sack of concrete in your hands. Well, the same thing holds true if you're overweight. When you stop growing and have reached your full height, your vertebrae have assumed a size (vertebral body diameter, pedicle diameter, facet surface area, lamina width) that's correct for that height. If you then put on an additional 30, 50, 80, or more pounds, your lumbar spine will be very unhappy and eventually cry out in pain. If you're 30, 50, or 80 pounds overweight, then it's as if you, too, are carrying around a sack of concrete weighing 30, 50, or 80 pounds— from the moment you get up in the morning until the moment you lie down in bed at night.

That extra weight does many things.

+ It shifts your weight-bearing line, or center of gravity, so that you have to extend (bend backward) all the time to keep from falling forward. This, in turn, puts extra pressure on the facet joints, compressing them and causing them to rub and wear: You develop facet joint arthritis.

+ It puts extra downward force on the lower lumbar discs, and they in turn have to work extra hard to push their adjacent vertebral bodies apart to maintain proper disc height.

+ As years pass, the discs lose the battle. The vertebral bodies push down so much with the force of your extra weight that the discs begin to narrow, the vertebral end plates begin to thicken, and you've got degenerative disc disease with disc bulging that may eventually turn into a disc herniation.

So use some sensible method to take off some, most, or all of those excess pounds. It always feels so good when you can put down a 30-, 50-, or 80-pound sack of concrete! Unfortunately, if some changes have already occurred, they're going to remain forever. But with the excess weight gone, the *progression* of these changes will markedly slow—and occasionally stop—and that's wonderful.

SMOKING

Does cigarette smoke cause herniated discs? No. Does it cause degenerative arthritis? No. So what's the big deal? The big deal is that smoking cigarettes is associated with high blood pressure and coronary artery disease. This bad, *bad* combination represents three very significant risk factors in the development of **atherosclerosis**, areas of fatty deposits on the inner walls of arteries that narrow them and constrict blood flow. The theory—which looks more and more correct the more we study the effects of smoking—is that damage caused by atherosclerosis to the blood vessels that supply the discs and facet joints is what leads to degenerative changes in the discs and facet joints. This, of course, compounds the damage caused by being overweight.

A study which was presented at the Sixty-Eighth Annual Meeting of the American Academy of Orthopaedic Surgeons in 2001 involved 1,337 doctors who graduated from the Johns Hopkins School of Medicine between 1948 and 1964. This was what is called a **prospective study** in which the subjects being examined are checked and their medical records reviewed year by year going forward, rather than reviewing their medical records from the past, a **retrospective study**. Some doctors were studied for as long as fifty-three years.

The prospective study allowed the researchers to determine whether the risk factors of smoking and high cholesterol came *before* the patients developed degenerative changes in their lumbar spines, or whether the degenerative changes came first, and the smoking and high cholesterol came later. You guessed it: The smoking and high cholesterol came first; the degenerative changes came later.

If you smoke, this is a good study to make you want to cut back drastically or to quit altogether. Again, cutting back or quitting won't undo changes that are already present, but it may reduce the rate at which more changes occur. That alone is worth it.

ALCOHOL

No scientific study has shown a direct link between alcohol consumption and degenerated or herniated discs or degenerative arthritis in the lumbar spine. This doesn't mean that you should go out and drink yourself into a stupor each night. The problem lies in the combination of excessive alcohol intake (more than two drinks a day on a regular basis) and lack of a proper nutritious diet, exercise, and so on. The excessive alcohol intake alone may lead to certain changes in the physiology of the body (how it takes in and metabolizes nutrients), which then can accelerate degenerative changes. Alcohol in moderation should have no ill effect on the spine.

CALCIUM

We learned in the last chapter that calcium is needed for bone growth and for bone maintenance. Calcium requirements change with age. Young children, for example, need about 800 milligrams of calcium a day, while preteens and adolescents ages nine through eighteen need between 1,200 and 1,500 milligrams of calcium per day. Between the ages of nineteen and fifty, you need 1,000 milligrams per day. After age fifty, you need 1,200 milligrams per day. These requirements are the same for both males and females at every age.

But remember that 99 percent of the calcium in the body is found in the bones, and only 1 percent is found in the bloodstream and elsewhere.

Also remember that women start losing calcium earlier in life than men, and women lose it at a faster rate than men until women are past menopause. So it's absolutely crucial that adolescent girls and young adult women get their full calcium intake daily as they grow and enter early adulthood, so that they have bones that are fully filled with calcium before age thirty. This doesn't mean that they—*or anyone at any age from nine to ninety*—should be taking *excessive* amounts of calcium daily, such as 2,000 milligrams or more; doing so does not promote more bone growth, but it may lead to kidney stones! The best way to try to prevent osteoporosis is to be certain to take the proper daily amount of calcium in your diet throughout childhood, adolescence, and early adulthood.

Good Sources of Calcium

It's easier than you think to increase your calcium intake. Just three to four servings each day of the foods listed below will add up to about 1,200 milligrams of calcium. Bon appétit!

Food	Amount of calcium
1 cup (8 oz.) nonfat milk	300 mg
1 cup (8 oz.) nonfat yogurt	300 mg
2 oz. nonfat cheese (2 slices)	300 mg
2 cups cottage cheese	400 mg
1 cup low-fat ice cream	190 mg
1 cup calcium-fortified orange juice	285 mg
1 slice calcium-fortified diet white bread	190 mg
1 slice calcium-fortified diet whole wheat bread	170 mg

CALCIUM CONTENT OF FOODS PER 100-GRAM PORTION (ABOUT 3.5 OUNCES)

Artichokes	51 mg
Beans (can: pinto, black)	135 mg
Beet greens (cooked)	99 mg
Black-eyed peas	55 mg
Broccoli (raw)	48 mg
Cauliflower (cooked)	42 mg
Chickpeas (garbanzos)	150 mg
Collards (raw leaves)	250 mg
Kale (raw leaves)	249 mg
Kale (cooked leaves)	187 mg
Lettuce (light green)	35 mg
Lettuce (dark green)	68 mg
Okra (raw or cooked)	92 mg
Olives	61 mg
Peanuts (roasted and salted)	74 mg
Peas (boiled)	56 mg
Pistachio nuts	131 mg
Raisins	62 mg
Rhubarb (cooked)	78 mg
Soybeans	60 mg
Spinach (raw)	93 mg
Swiss chard (raw)	88 mg
Tofu	128 mg

Turnip greens (raw)	246 mg
Turnip greens (boiled)	184 mg
Watercress	151 mg

VITAMIN D

It will do you no good to take the proper amount of calcium for your age if you don't also take vitamin D. It's the vitamin D that actually arranges for the calcium in your blood to get into the bone: No vitamin D—no calcium transport into bone. The amount needed is the same for both sexes. Children, adolescents, and adults up to age fifty need 200 IU (international units) of vitamin D per day. Adults ages fifty to sixty-nine need 400 IU per day. Those seventy and older need 600 IU per day. One glass of vitamin-D-enriched milk contains 400 IU. Twenty minutes of bright sunshine will create the same amount. It's important to realize that, for sunlight to help the body make vitamin D, you can't have on sunblock. If you're out and about doing errands and the like, there's a good chance you'll get twenty minutes of sunshine in the summer without wearing sunblock. Of course, you don't want to get skin cancer, so be careful!

REGULAR EXERCISE

In chapter 5, you learned that low-impact aerobic exercises can help in the rehabilitation of back injuries. These same exercises are also excellent for helping condition the back and keep it and the paraspinal muscles in shape. Walking is wonderful, dancing is ducky, and jogging is just great. They're all weight-bearing exercises—which is what makes them good. Anyone at any age can begin a walking program. Those who are more physically fit can jog. (Others should check with their doctors and build up gradually.) Sports such as tennis, golf (walking the course, not using a cart), and handball are excellent. Swimming will help strengthen the paraspinal muscles but not the bones. To be effective, your exercise program should be done at least three times a week (more, if you can) for at least thirty to sixty minutes each time.

POSTURE

Mom always told you, "Sit up straight!" and "Hold your head high when you walk!" As always, she was right. When you sit, sit back in the chair; use a small rolled towel or pillow at the low lumbar region, if necessary; use a chair with a high enough back support; and make sure it's the proper height so your feet are flat on the floor. Wear shoes with heels no higher than 1.5 inches (4 centimeters) and try to avoid flat shoes with virtually no heels. Shoes of the proper height allow you to stand easily with weight properly transmitted down your spine and across your pelvis and hips. The lumbar lordotic curve will be correct, and your back won't ache from prolonged standing. Try to keep briefcases and the like from being overloaded so you don't create a long lever arm that alters your posture. The same holds true for backpacks: They can be especially harmful to proper back posture and dynamics if they're overloaded!

Strange as it seems, sometimes going barefoot can increase backache by causing the weight bearing line to shift from its ideal alignment. This then changes the dynamics of how forces are transmitted from head to spine to hips to feet, and lower back pain results!

If you must stand for prolonged periods, do what I told pregnant women to do: Get a small footstool and alternate placing one foot on it. This is a simple yet very effective way to keep good posture while standing. And when you lie down to sleep, your best posture will occur when you're either on your back or on your side. A pillow between your knees while side-lying keeps your legs and pelvis aligned.

BENDING, LIFTING, AND CARRYING

When you pick up something from below waist height, bend your knees and lift with your legs while keeping your back straight. Don't bend at the waist and then lift by straightening up. Also, when you lift, go to great lengths to avoid simultaneous bending, lifting, and twisting. Carry things close to you, not with outstretched arms, to avoid the sharp increase in the force that will be transmitted to the lower lumbar discs.

SPECIAL BACK EXERCISES

Do you recall those stretching and strengthening exercises for the back muscles and the abdominal muscles that I described in chapters 5 and 8 as helpful in the treatment of lower back pain? Well, guess what? They're also really good for keeping the back in shape and for trying to prevent back pain in the first place. Those home exercises really are easy to do, don't take very long, and are a simple, effective way of maintaining back flexibility and back and abdominal muscle strength and tone. The prone and standing extension, sitting and supine flexion, sitting flexion to extension, and bicycle mini sit-ups are just the ticket to staying in good shape.

Wow! We did it! We accomplished everything that we set out to do. We've learned all about the lumbar spine, what it is, how it works, what happens when it goes bad, how we figure out what went wrong, what we can do to make it better, and how we can try to keep it in good shape. Now if we hear someone tell us to keep our feet firmly on the ground, our head in the clouds, our shoulder to the wheel, our nose to the grindstone, and then try working in that position, we'll know that we can do it and still avoid hurting. I can't resist saying it: I think we all should give ourselves a pat on the back!

Glossary

acute: coming on suddenly, and lasting up to six months

annulus fibrosus: the outer, thick gristle ring of an intervertebral disc

anterior longitudinal ligament: the ligament connecting the fronts of all of the vertebral bodies; it is closest to the abdominal cavity in the lumbar region

anterior: toward the front of a bone or the body

apposing: the term applied to two bony surfaces that face each other

arthritis: the condition that results from the microtrauma-caused wear and tear of bones, ligaments, and joints

artificial disc implantation: a relatively new and still experimental surgical procedure in which an intervertebral disc is removed and replaced by metal plates containing a synthetic material to mimic the disc

assessment: comparison by the doctor of subjective patient complaints with objective findings on physical examination

atherosclerosis: a disease of arteries in which cholesterol deposits, or plaques, form

automated percutaneous microdiscectomy: a surgical procedure in which miniaturized instruments are inserted through a tiny incision, with guidance from a videofluoroscope, to remove the intervertebral disc using a tiny motorized grinder; the ligamentum flavum, paraspinal muscles, and lumbodorsal fascia are not cut into or removed

autotraction: a treatment technique in which the body's own weight is used to create a distracting pull across the vertebrae to pull them apart.

back brace: a rigid device worn externally that limits motion in a portion of the spine

bilateral: on both sides of a vertebra

bilateral spondylolysis: absence of bone in both partes interarticulares of a vertebra; it can lead to spondylolisthesis

body: the cylindrical, frontmost, main part of a vertebra

bone density: a measure of the concentration and amount of calcium in bone

bone scan: a picture of a part of the body created by a type of Geiger counter called a gamma camera, after a minute quantity of radioactive dye has been injected into the bloodstream

bulging disc: a protruding intervertebral disc that does not impinge upon or indent the thecal sac and/or spinal nerve root

capillaries: the tiniest ends of arteries that bring nutrients to individual tissues and dilate in response to the application of heat

cartilage: the ultrasmooth tissue covering the end of a bone to create the surface of a joint

CAT: the acronym for computerized axial tomography

CAT scan: a computer-generated x-ray of a cross section of part of the body, which can show bones, muscles, and intervertebral discs with good detail

cauda equina: the spinal nerve roots that continue down through the spinal canal below the first lumbar vertebra where the spinal cord itself ends

cervical vertebra: one of the seven neck bones

chemonucleolysis: a surgical procedure in which a needle is inserted into the intervertebral disc and the disc is dissolved with an enzyme called chymopapain

chief complaint: the reason for seeing the doctor

chronic: lasting more than six months

coccyx: the tailbone consisting of four tiny bones at the lower end of the spine

codfish vertebra: a condition in which osteoporosis weakens the vertebral end plate so much that the stronger intervertebral disc pushes the vertebral end plate into the body of the vertebra, making it look like a codfish on an x-ray

cold thermoreceptor: the tiny skin nerve ending that senses cold; it does not change the temperature of the skin

compression fracture: a fracture causing a wedge-shaped deformity of the body of a vertebra

congenital anomaly: a bony condition that is present at birth and is usually not hereditary

cortex: the dense, hard, outer part of a bone

deep friction massage: a physical therapy technique in which the therapist applies very strong pressure to the skin transverse to the direction of muscle fibers; also called transverse friction massage

degenerative disc disease: a chronic condition in which the loss of water in the nucleus pulposus of an intervertebral disc results in loss of disc height, usually with reactive changes in the vertebral end plates and/or the anterior and posterior longitudinal ligaments

degenerative scoliosis: curvature of the spine that occurs when asymmetric degeneration of an intervertebral disc causes tilting of the vertebra above it

degenerative spondylolisthesis: forward slipping of one vertebra in relation to the vertebra below, caused by severe bilateral degeneration of the slipping vertebra's facet joints

dermatome: the longitudinal band of sensation supplied by one spinal nerve root

discogram: an x-ray that shows an intervertebral disc after a special dye has been injected into the disc

distensibility: the stretchability of muscle tissue

double-blind study: a scientific study in which neither the person being treated nor the doctor evaluating the treatment knows whether an actual medication/treatment or a placebo has been used

dynamic stabilization exercises: a physical therapy technique for strengthening the back muscles by training them in the least painful position, called the neutral position

electromyogram: a test in which needle electrodes are inserted into a muscle to measure its electrical activity during rest and while it contracts; abnormal electrical activity means that there is irritation of the spinal nerve root supplying the muscle

epidural fat: a special globular fatty tissue attached to the surface of the thecal sac covering the spinal nerve roots; it can act as a buffer between the thecal sac and the intervertebral disc below it

extension: the motion of straightening up from a bent forward position, or bending backward beyond the straight position

facet: a projection from a lamina or pedicle

facet joint: the joint where motion occurs between one vertebra and the next

femoral nerve: a nerve trunk formed by spinal nerve roots from the upper lumbar vertebrae; it comes around the pelvis to supply all the muscles and skin of the front of the thigh

flexion exercises: a physical therapy technique for strengthening the abdominal muscles

flexion: the motion of bending forward from a straight position

free fragment: a piece of herniated intervertebral disc that has broken off and is lying loose in the spinal canal, usually causing severe pressure on a nerve root or the thecal sac

hemisacralization: a transitional fifth lumbar vertebra that has failed to segment completely on one side only, has one enlarged transverse process, and has taken on the appearance of a first sacral vertebra on that side

herniated disc: a protruding intervertebral disc that impinges upon or indents the thecal sac and/or spinal nerve root; lay synonyms include slipped disc and chipped disc

high voltage galvanic stimulation: a physical therapy modality that is a type of electrical stimulation to make muscles contract and relax repeatedly; also called microdyne

history: chronologic story describing an injury from the time it occurred to the time of examination

hypertrophy: thickening or enlarging of a bone in response to stress forces

ilium: the big hip bone on each side of the pelvis that connects to the sacrum

inflammatory stage: the first of the three stages of soft-tissue healing, which lasts from a few days to two weeks

inspection: visually examining, or looking at, an area at the start of the physical examination

interbody fusion: a surgical procedure in which an intervertebral disc is removed, and a device is inserted in its place, containing bone or other material that will unite with the vertebral body above and below it to make a solid unit

interspinous ligament: the ligament connecting one vertebral spinous process to the next

intertransverse ligament: the ligament connecting one vertebral transverse process to the next

intervertebral disc: the shock-absorbing cushion between each pair of vertebrae

intervertebral foramen: the opening ("window") bounded by adjacent pedicles through which exits a spinal nerve root; also called a neural foramen

joint: the articulation where two bones meet

kyphosis: the C-shaped curve seen in the midback when a person is viewed from the side; the midpart of the C faces toward the back of the body

lamina: half of the roof of a vertebra; it also serves as the roof of the spinal canal

laminae: the Latin plural for *lamina*

laminectomy: a surgical procedure in which a long skin incision is made in the back, the ligamentum flavum is removed, and the intervertebral disc is excised

ligament: a dense gristle tissue that connects one bone to another and acts as a hinge or stabilizer

ligamentum flavum: the "yellow ligament" that connects one vertebral lamina to the next; it also serves as the roof of the spinal canal

lordosis: the C-shaped curve seen in the neck and low back when a person is viewed from the side; the midpart of the C faces toward the front (the stomach in the lumbar region)

lumbar microdiscectomy: a surgical procedure similar to a standard laminectomy, but using a very short skin incision; the ligamentum flavum is still removed, and the intervertebral disc is excised

lumbar pain: lower back pain in pregnant women, related to prolonged sitting, standing, walking, and carrying

lumbar vertebra: one of the five bones of the low back

lumbarization: a transitional first sacral vertebra that has segmented and taken on the appearance of a lumbar vertebra

lumbodorsal fascia: a tough gristle tissue that surrounds and contains the paraspinal muscles, separating them from the subcutaneous fat

manual muscle examination: formal testing of the strength of an individual muscle

massage: a physical therapy technique in which the therapist's hands and fingers knead the back muscles

McKenzie extension exercises: a physical therapy technique for strengthening the posterior paraspinal muscles

microtrauma: microscopic injuries to individual bone cells, ligaments, tendons, and muscles that result in the leaking of individual blood cells

modalities: physical therapy techniques including heat, ice, ultrasound, and high-voltage galvanic stimulation (microdyne)

MRI: the acronym for magnetic resonance imaging

MRI scan: a computer-generated magnetic picture of a longitudinal section, cross section, or frontal section of a part of the body that shows bones, muscles, ligaments, discs, nerves, arteries, and veins with good detail; it is *not* an x-ray

muscle: a specialized soft tissue that can only contract or shorten; it connects two bones and creates motion by contracting

muscle relaxant: a prescription medication that may reduce muscle spasm by causing skeletal muscles, especially the paraspinal muscles, to relax

myelogram: an x-ray that shows the spinal cord and spinal nerve roots after a special dye has been injected inside their covering; indentation of the dye implies pressure from an intervertebral disc and / or bone spur

nerve conduction test: a test in which surface electrodes measure the speed and quality of electrical impulses transmitted by a nerve; abnormal electrical activity means that there is irritation of the spinal nerve root from which the nerve derives

neural arch: the name applied to the laminae during fetal development

neurologic extremity examination: an examination testing the legs for sensation, motor power, and reflexes

NSAID: the acronym for nonsteroidal anti-inflammatory drug, an arthritis medicine not containing cortisone, or steroid.

nucleus pulposus: the central, spongy part of an intervertebral disc

objective: the findings of the doctor during a physical examination

objective finding: something that is beyond a patient's control, such as an x-ray

orthopaedic extremity examination: inspection, palpation, range of motion, and manual muscle examination of the legs

orthopaedist: synonym for orthopaedic surgeon, a doctor who treats bones, muscles, joints, tendons, ligaments, and the bones and discs of the spine by both surgical and nonsurgical techniques

osteoblasts: cells that make bone

osteoclasts: cells that break down bone

osteoporosis: a condition in which resorption of bone exceeds bone formation

palpation: using the fingertips to feel for areas of tenderness or spasm

paraspinal muscles: the muscles that connect the vertebrae together and by contracting, or shortening, either pull them upright, bend them to the right or left, or rotate or twist them

paresthesias: a feeling of pins and needles, or tingling

pedicle: a pillar projecting backward from the body of a vertebra; it also serves as the side of the spinal canal

pedicle screw: a screw inserted through a vertebral pedicle, usually serving as an anchor for spinal instrumentation such as plates or rods

percussion: tapping an area to see if pain is elicited

physical examination: a doctor's hands-on examination of a patient; it consists of inspection, palpation, percussion, range of motion, orthopaedic, and neurologic tests

physical therapy: a type of treatment that is used externally and involves a variety of mechanical means to try to heal structures deep inside the body

pinched nerve: the lay term for a herniated disc pressing on a spinal nerve and causing nerve root irritation including radiating pain, paresthesias, and/or numbness

placebo: a sham or fake medicine or treatment

plan: treatment program devised by the doctor, which is based on the diagnosis following the history and physical examination

plane x-ray: a flat, two-dimensional picture of a part of the body showing only structures that contain calcium, such as bones

posterior longitudinal ligament: the ligament connecting the backs of all the vertebral bodies; it also serves as the floor of the spinal canal

posterior pelvic pain: pain in the back at the waistline in pregnant women, which goes down to the back, and possibly the front, of the pelvis

posterior spine fusion: a surgical procedure in which a long skin incision is made in the back, the paraspinal muscles are detached, and bone is placed across the back side of the laminae

posterior spine fusion with instrumentation: a surgical procedure in which a standard posterior spine fusion is combined with the attachment of rods, plates, and/or pedicle screws

posterior: toward the back of a bone or the body

proliferative stage: the second of the three stages of soft-tissue healing, which begins around the third day after an injury

prospective study: a scientific study that analyzes data collected from patients beginning with the date the study starts and going forward in time

radiculopathy: irritation along the course of a spinal nerve root; it may be manifested as radiating pain, paresthesias, and/or numbness

randomized double-blind study: a scientific study in which patients are randomly assigned to receive either an actual medication/treatment or a placebo and in which neither the person being treated nor the doctor evaluating the treatment knows whether an actual medication/treatment or a placebo has been used

range of motion: measurement of the ability to flex, extend, side bend, and rotate

reactive sclerosis: extra bone that forms as a reaction to the slowly propagating fracture line of a stress fracture

relaxin: a hormone found in pregnant women that causes muscles and ligaments to relax

remodeling stage: the third of the three stages of soft-tissue healing, which continues for about six weeks after an injury

resorption: the breaking down of bone with loss of its calcium

retrospective study: a scientific study that analyzes data collected in the past from patients prior to the date the study started

sacralization: a transitional fifth lumbar vertebra that has failed to segment completely, has enlarged transverse processes, and has taken on the appearance of a first sacral vertebra

sacroiliac belt: a wide, flat, mildly elastic belt that goes around the body at the upper part of the ilium bones and helps to compress them against the sacrum

sacroiliac ligament: a dense, tough ligament that connects the sacrum to the ilium bone

sacrum: the base of the spine, consisting of five fused vertebrae

sciatic nerve: a thick nerve trunk formed by spinal nerve roots from the lower lumbar spine and sacrum. It goes down the back of the thigh and calf and supplies the muscles of the back of the thigh and all the muscles of the calf, ankle, and foot as well as the skin of the back of the thigh and all skin below the knee

sciatic shift: a shift to the left or right in the low back caused by intense muscle spasm, seen in an acute low back strain

sciatica: pain along the course of the sciatic nerve

scoliosis: curvature of the spine as viewed from behind a person; it can be C-shaped or S-shaped

segmental spasm: replacement of the normal lumbar smooth side-bending curve by what appears to be two straight lines that bend at one point, as a result of muscle spasm seen in an acute low back strain

segmentation: the separating of neural tissue into discrete vertebrae that occurs around the sixth to eighth week of fetal development

semi-Fowler's position: the reclining chair position, which helps relieve back pain

side bending: the motion of tilting to the right or left at the waist

SOAP: the acronym for subjective, objective, assessment, plan, which describes the way a doctor's office notes are organized

soft tissues: muscles, ligaments, tendons, and intervertebral discs

spinal canal: the central, open area of a vertebra through which the spinal cord and spinal nerve roots travel; its floor is the posterior longitudinal ligament, its walls are the pedicles, and its roof is the ligamentum flavum and laminae

spinal claudication: pain in the leg(s) and/or buttock(s) when the back is extended, often seen in spinal stenosis (and it has nothing to do with vascular claudication); it's also called neurogenic claudication

spinal stenosis: narrowing of the spinal canal, caused by a combination of bulging of the intervertebral disc and posterior longitudinal ligament, and hypertrophy of the pedicles, laminae, and ligamentum flavum

spine fusion: a surgical procedure that removes all motion at an area of the spine

spinous process: a projection extending backward from the area where two laminae join

spondylolisthesis: forward slipping of one vertebra in relation to the vertebra below, caused by bilateral spondylolysis

spondylolysis: absence of bone in the pars interarticularis, which may occur on one or both sides of a vertebra

sprain: an injury to a muscle

spur: an outward bony projection usually occurring as a result of repeated microtrauma over a prolonged period of time; synonyms are hypertrophic spur and bone spur

strain: an injury to a ligament

strengthening exercises: a physical therapy technique for improving muscle tone and strength

stress fracture: a very slowly occurring fracture caused by the gradual weakening of a bone from frequently repeated stresses

stretching exercises: a physical therapy technique for overcoming muscle tightness

subcutaneous fat: the fatty tissue under the skin

subjective: the patient's perception of what seems to be wrong, as related to the doctor who is taking the history

subjective response: something that is completely under the control of the patient, such as a complaint of pain when a body part is touched, and that cannot be verified by a specific scientific test

synovium: the special soft tissue that surrounds and encloses a joint

TENS: the acronym for transcutaneous electric nerve stimulation

TENS unit: a battery-powered device that sends electric signals through the skin, supposedly to overwhelm and block the transmission of pain nerve impulses from the back to the brain

thecal sac: the covering of the spinal cord and spinal nerve roots

thoracic vertebra: one of the twelve midback bones to which the ribs attach

traction: a treatment technique in which weights are attached to a harness at the waist or on the legs in an attempt to distract, or pull apart, the vertebrae

transcutaneous: across or through the skin

transitional vertebra: a vertebra in which some parts are formed incompletely or excessively, resulting in either partial or complete lumbarization or sacralization

transverse process: a projection extending out from the side of the pedicle of a vertebra; also, in the thoracic spine, the place where a rib attaches

trigger point: a discrete, tiny area of sharp, intense pain in muscle or gristle tissue

trigger point injection: an injection usually containing a local anesthetic plus cortisone, which is infiltrated into a trigger point

ultrasound: a physical therapy modality consisting of high-frequency sound waves that create heat; it's also called therapeutic ultrasound to distinguish it from diagnostic ultrasound, which is used, for example, to determine fetal size in pregnancy

unilateral: on one side of a vertebra

unilateral spondylolysis: the absence of bone in one pars interarticularis of a vertebra

vacuum disc phenomenon: the replacement of the water content of an intervertebral disc by nitrogen gas as a result of severe degeneration of the disc

vascular claudication: cramping in the calves caused by poor arterial circulation; it has nothing to do with spinal claudication

vertebra: one of the thirty-three bones that forms the spine

vertebrae: the Latin plural for vertebra

vertebral end plate: the flat surface of the end of a vertebral body that abuts against the intervertebral disc

water exercises: aerobic back exercises performed in a pool

weight-bearing line: a line, from head to feet, that passes through the center of gravity just in front of the spine

Quick Review Guide

SPRAIN/STRAIN

Symptoms

Onset of pain, limited motion, and stiffness within hours or days after a particular activity. Pain increases with activity and is relieved by rest.

Physical Examination

Loss of lordosis, possible sciatic shift, decreased motion, spasm. Normal neurologic examination.

Lumbar Spine X-rays

Normal

Treatment

Ice, NSAIDs, physical therapy

SACROILIAC SPRAIN/STRAIN

Symptoms

Onset of pain, limited motion, and stiffness at the sacroiliac joint, usually within hours after a particular activity. Pain increases with activity and when rolling over while lying down. Sometimes accompanied by ipsilateral leg pain.

Physical Examination

Intense pain directly over sacroiliac joint, limited motion, sometimes spasm. Normal neurologic examination.

Lumbar Spine X-rays	Normal
MRI scan, CAT scan	Normal
EMGs and NCTs	Normal
Treatment	Ice, NSAIDs, home sacroiliac stretching exercises, Sacroiliac belt, physical therapy

FACET JOINT IRRITATION

Symptoms	Gradual onset usually after bending, twisting, lifting, etc. Pain increases with activity and when rolling over while lying down. Sometimes accompanied by ipsilateral leg pain.
Physical Examination	Intense pain directly over irritated lumbar facet, limited motion, sometimes spasm, sciatic shift. Normal neurologic examination.
Lumbar Spine X-rays	Usually normal. May show a rotated facet joint.
MRI scan, CAT scan	Normal
EMGs and NCTs	Normal
Treatment	NSAIDs, physical therapy. If symptoms persist for more than 6 to 8 weeks, video-fluoroscopic-guided facet joint injection.

HERNIATED DISC (PINCHED NERVE)

Symptoms	Rapid onset of back pain, radiating leg pain, paresthesias and numbness after lifting, bending, carrying, etc. Sometimes a feeling of leg weakness.
Physical Examination	Limited motion, possible sciatic shift, spasm, abnormal neurologic examination with changes possible in sensation, motor power, reflex
Lumbar Spine X-rays	Normal
MRI scan, CAT scan	Herniated disc
Lumbar Myelogram	Herniated disc
Lumbar Discogram	May show herniated disc (not as reliable as other studies)
EMGs and NCTs	Abnormal
Treatment	Surgery is almost always necessary.

COMPRESSION FRACTURE

Symptoms	Rapid onset of pain after falling, jumping, or other injury. Pain often intense, even at rest, and usually localized to fractured area.
Physical Examination	Tenderness often localized, spasm, limited motion. Neurologic examination usually normal.
Lumbar Spine X-rays	Compression fracture
MRI scan, CAT scan	Compression fracture

Three-phase Bone Scan	Compression fracture
EMGs and NCTs	Normal

PAINFUL COCCYX

Symptoms	Rapid onset of pain after falling and landing on buttocks; also during childbirth.
Physical Examination	Exquisite tenderness over coccyx and normal neurologic examination
Lumbar Spine X-rays	Fractured coccyx
Treatment	Rolled towel behind knee when sitting, NSAIDs, physical therapy including whirlpool

DEGENERATIVE ARTHRITIS

Symptoms	Pain may be constant or intermittent, and it may be mild, moderate, or severe. Pain may increase with activities and subside with rest.
Physical Examination	Stiffness, reduced motion, sometimes loss of lordosis and pain during motion and neurologic examination normal
Lumbar Spine X-rays	Spurring of facets and/or pedicles
MRI scan, CAT scan	Bony spurring; spurs do not impinge on nerve roots or thecal sac.
EMGs and NCTs	Normal
Treatment	NSAIDs, home exercises, physical therapy, water (pool) therapy

DEGENERATIVE DISC DISEASE

Symptoms

Pain may be constant or intermittent, and it may be mild, moderate, or severe. Pain may increase with activities and subside with rest, and sometimes it may go into one or both legs.

Physical Examination

Possibly tenderness or limited motion, motion accompanied by pain, sometimes segmental spasm, and neurologic examination usually normal

Lumbar Spine X-rays

Narrowing of the intervertebral disc space. Often bone spurs and thickening of the vertebral end plates.

MRI scan

Loss of water in the disc, narrowing of the intervertebral disc space, bulging of the disc, bone spurs, vertebral end plate thickening. May sometimes show nerve root impingement.

EMGs and NCTs

Abnormal if nerve root impingement is present.

Treatment

NSAIDs, physical therapy, aerobic and water (pool) exercises, home exercises and moist heat if no evidence of nerve root impingement

SPINAL STENOSIS

Symptoms

Constant, dull, unremitting backache, constant or intermittent radiating leg pain, paresthesias, numbness, spinal claudication

Physical Examination	Pain on extension often accompanied by paresthesias and numbness, restricted motion, neurologic examination may be abnormal.
Lumbar Spine X-rays	Bony spurring of vertebral end plates, pedicles, foramina, and laminae
MRI scan, CAT scan	Same as x-rays plus thickening of ligamentum flavum, bulging or herniated discs, indentation of thecal sac, possible nerve root impingement.
Myelogram	Indentation or kinking of thecal sac
EMGs and NCTs	May show abnormalities
Treatment	NSAIDs, physical therapy, aerobic and water (pool) exercises. Avoid McKenzie exercises. Surgery may be necessary if symptoms persist or progress.

STRESS FRACTURE

Symptoms	Gradual onset of intermittent pain, which eventually becomes continuous. Pain increases with activity and decreases with rest.
Physical Examination	Spasm, tenderness, possible segmental spasm. Neurologic examination is normal.
Lumbar Spine X-rays	Early: normal Later: reactive sclerosis, fracture line
MRI scan, CAT scan	Early: stress fracture
Three-phase Bone Scan	Best test. Early: stress fracture
EMGs and NCTs	Normal
Treatment	Back brace for 12 weeks

SPONDYLOLYSIS

Symptoms	Vague, usually intermittent lower back pain but may be constant, usually not increased by activity.
Physical Examination	Localized tenderness, possible spasm, normal motion. Neurologic examination is normal.
Lumbar Spine X-rays	Spondylolysis
MRI scan, CAT scan	Spondylolysis
EMGs and NCTs	Normal
Treatment	Back brace sometimes, physical therapy, NSAIDs

SPONDYLOLISTHESIS

Symptoms	Often painless. Sometimes constant pain, occasionally leg pain, tight hamstrings.
Physical Examination	Step-off on palpation, tight hamstrings
Lumbar Spine X-rays	Spondylolisthesis
MRI scan, CAT scan	Spondylolisthesis. Will show extent of disc protrusion.
EMGs and NCTs	Usually normal
Treatment	Trial of physical therapy in patients with minimal slipping. Spine fusion is usually required.

TRANSITIONAL VERTEBRAE
(LUMBARIZATION, SACRALIZATION)

Symptoms

Pain at lumbo-sacral junction, sometimes radiating leg pain

Physical Examination

Possible loss of lordosis, sciatic shift, spasm. Severe tenderness over abnormality, limited motion.

Lumbar Spine X-rays

Transitional vertebra

Treatment

Physical therapy, NSAIDs, home exercises. Rarely: surgery to fuse transitional vertebrae

Sudden Acute Lower Back Pain

AREA OF PAIN:	POSSIBLE CONDITION:
Midline Lumbar	Sprain/Strain* / Herniated Disc / Compression Fracture Painful Coccyx / Facet Joint Irritation
Lateral Lumbar	Sprain/Strain* / Facet Joint Irritation
Sacroiliac (Lateral)	Sacroiliac Sprain/Strain*
Coccyx (Midline)	Painful Coccyx
No Radiating Leg Pain	Sprain/Strain* / Compression Fracture Painful Coccyx / Facet Joint Irritation / Sacroiliac Sprain/Strain / Painful Coccyx
Pain Radiating into the Leg	Sprain/Strain* / Herniated Disc / Facet Joint Irritation / Sacroiliac Sprain/Strain
No Radiating Leg Pain, but with Pseudo Pins and Needles/Numbness	Sprain/Strain* / Facet Joint Irritation / Sacroiliac Sprain/Strain
Radiating Leg Pain with Pins and Needles/Numbness	Herniated Disc

* May or may not cause radiating leg pain.

Gradually-Occurring Lower Back Pain

AREA OF PAIN:	**POSSIBLE CONDITION:**
Midline Lumbar	Degenerative Disc Disease / Degenerative Arthritis / Spinal Stenosis / Spondylolysis / Spondylolisthesis / Degenerative Spondylolisthesis
Lateral Lumbar	Degenerative Disc Disease / Degenerative Arthritis / Spinal Stenosis / Spondylolysis / Spondylolisthesis / Degenerative Spondylolisthesis / Stress Fracture
Sacroiliac	Transitional Vertebra
No Radiating Leg Pain	Degenerative Arthritis / Spondylolysis / Stress Fracture / Transitional Vertebra
Radiating Leg Pain without Pins and Needles/Numbness	Degenerative Disc Disease / Degenerative Arthritis / Spondylolisthesis / Degenerative Spondylolisthesis / Transitional Vertebra / Stress Fracture
Radiating Leg Pain with Pins and Needles/Numbness	Degenerative Disc Disease / Spondylolisthesis / Degenerative Spondylolisthesis / Spinal Stenosis

Index